In My Own Words:
Women's Experience of Hysterectomy

Published by the Hysterectomy Association

Edited by Linda Parkinson-Hardman

for Claire Edge

Thankyou & best wishes

Linda ☺

Copyright

First edition published 31st July 2013

By: the Hysterectomy Association

ISBN: 978-0-9532445-6-0

British Library Cataloguing in Publication Data. A catalogue record for this book is available from The British Library.

Telephone: 0843 289 2142

Website: www.hysterectomy-association.org.uk

Cover Image: © Rmarmion, Alexander Chistyakov, Yuri Arcurs at Dreamstime.com

Disclaimer

Although much of this book represents current medical opinion, some of the information and resources listed by story contributors are by definition, outside the scope of generally accepted medical standards of care. They may be non-conventional, alternative or complementary. The information and resources listed should not be used in any way to provide a diagnosis or to prescribe any medical treatment. As in the case of conventional medicine, indiscriminate use of some therapies presented, without medical supervision, may be harmful to your health. Individuals reading this material should, in all cases, consult their own doctor or health practitioner for the diagnosis and treatment of medical conditions. The author and publisher cannot accept responsibility for illness arising out of failure to seek medical advice from a doctor.

Acknowledgements

This book would not have come about without the support of a great many people. Many of them funded the book directly through a crowd-funded project that took place on Kickstarter in early 2013; others supported it by sharing the project details and their enthusiasm for the book on their websites, blogs and social accounts like Facebook and Twitter.

In total 85 people funded this book; my thanks and those of the women it will help go to each and every one of them. Special thanks go in particular to:

Elizabeth Harrison,
Margaret Griffin,
Mary Ruth,
Carol E Wyer,
Mike Little,
Purvi Kothari,
Clare Hackman,
Simo Muinonen,
Menna Williams,
Claire Edge,
Susannah Goss
Beth Caswell
Steve Graham of www.Internet-Mentor.co.uk
www.winahomefor life.com.

Thank you all so much, without you and your faith the book wouldn't be available for women in the future.

I'd also like to say a big thank you to Yvonne at Inbox Editorial Services for her astute and sensitive editing of the original stories; she helped them come to life with her suggestions and improvements for layout.

Finally, I need to share my gratitude to Carol Bentley, Anne Orchard, Robyn Chausse, Carole E Wyer, Mohana Rajakumar, Marc Nash, Madison Woods, Karen Dash, Destiny Allison, Denise M Hartman,

Matthew Hirtes, Chrissie Sainsbury, Deone Higgs Ashley McCook, Simo Muinonen, Anne Cooper, Yasmin Selena Butt, Westrow Cooper, Annie McDowall, Mark Blunden, Mike Little, Madison Woods, Lawrence Ainsworth, Lesley Fletcher, Women on the Verge, Hormones Matter, The Fertility and Infertility Research News Portal, First Post, The Sali Hoe Foundation for Cervical Cancer, Med Helper, Lucine Women Community. All of these people and organisations helped to spread the word about the project and allowed me to connect with their network of contacts too.

But perhaps the biggest thanks of all need to go to those women who have written their stories for the benefit of others. Without them and their willingness to share both the happiness and the sadness there would be no book.

Contents

This book is dedicated to Jess - thank you.

Introduction

Back in 1994 I had a hysterectomy; it wasn't a bad experience and to tell the truth I came through it all really well. I never had any really negative experiences and have never regretted the decision I made.

However, in 1997 I founded the Hysterectomy Association because I realised that despite being reasonably intelligent (or so I thought), I hadn't received the information I needed to make a fully informed choice. Since then the website has provided information and support to millions of women.

Over the last 15 years I've heard and read the stories of thousands of women who have used the website to talk to me and their comrades in health. They have told me about their experiences in ways that are unique to them but which have common threads and themes running through each one.

In 2007 I began collecting these stories together with the intention of using them to empower other women, probably in a book. The stories share loss, happiness, joy and pain; they speak of family and friends and isolation; they talk of the need to share with others who have been there, before they too can move on. This is not something which happens in many other surgical situations; it seems that having a hysterectomy really does cut to the heart of what being a woman is all about.

In the UK alone, around 38,000 women have a hysterectomy on the NHS every year and it's estimated that a further 20,000 take place in private hospitals. In the United States roughly 600,000 women will go through the procedure for reasons that vary from cancer to complications at child birth and fibroids to endometriosis and prolapse; it is the most commonly performed operation on women the world over.

I know from my experience running the Hysterectomy Association that other people's stories are profoundly important; they help women feel less isolated; they show that they aren't going mad, missing the point or stupid; they demonstrate that their concerns are genuine and real and that the only way to deal with them is to voice them.

There are 82 stories in this book. Each one is unique and will help at least one other woman to understand their experience better. They have been loosely divided into three sections, Before, During and After and have been very gently edited as the intention was to preserve as much of the natural voice of each writer; after all we each have our own way of expressing ourselves and our feelings and who am I to say that how one person says something is better than another's.

Some of the stories here are very short; they are snippets, glimpses into one woman's world and perspective; others are much longer, reading over several pages. A couple are written over more than one section because they are a progression - these should be obvious. You will also notice that there are a variety of naming conventions, some women preferred to remain anonymous, others shared their first name and even more their full name.

The majority of the stories are positive, but there are some negative and even quite harrowing ones but that is rare (as are the complications they speak of, thankfully). Hysterectomy doesn't have just one face, it has many and every one deserves to be seen.

At the back you will find a complete glossary of the terminology used throughout. Women who have been through the process, joined in the forums, shared on the website or on our Facebook page will recognise some of the acronyms and shorthand used, those who haven't yet made it there probably won't.

Whilst I would suggest that you read all the stories as they all have useful nuggets of information and support, I know that as humans we will always prefer to hear about the things that are closest to the situation we find ourselves in. Therefore I have included a list at the back of the stories categorised by subject, so you can jump in and find the right ones without having to read all if you prefer.

If, at the end of the book, you have found it helpful then why not let us and others know by leaving a review on the site you bought it from. Every positive review will help someone else to find them in the future too.

BEFORE

Thank You! Michelle Dobson

Four weeks ago I Googled hysterectomy,

That day I was feeling low,

Full of worry and apprehension

Due to continual menstrual flow!

This website appeared in front of me

But little did I know,

Just how much it would help

And the 'friendships' that would grow!

I clicked the link, wondering

Would this website suffice?

But got the most amazing welcome

Information and advice!

Those ladies on the 'done couch'

Quickly showed me the way

Offering so much support

And top tips every single day!

I then met other ladies

In the 'waiting room' too

And to have shared my journey with them

Well... I feel privileged, I do!

Every lady has a different story to tell,
That's personal to them and unique
And posting our experiences on here
Is a fantastic coping technique!

Pre-op I was overwhelmed,
with your messages of support,
And as I waited at the hospital
That was a very comforting thought!

When I landed on the 'done couch'
Rather bumpily...
Everyone was waiting
To support and congratulate me!

In the days that followed
I had a rough time
But so many lovely ladies
Kept making sure I was fine!

I'm 12 days post-op today
And want to say huge thanks
To everyone who's supporting me in recovery and just to say... that
'Googling hysterectomy' that day, made for an amazing discovery!

Very Frightened, Lizzy

In two weeks I am due to have a hysterectomy and also removal of a TVTO mesh tape! I am extremely scared. I have joined a support group for the mesh removal and hoped to find some comfort and support here as I know many ladies here have either had the operation or are about to undertake it.

My consultant cannot be 100% sure whether both the tape and the womb are causing the pain and problems. My womb is very enlarged and 10 years ago I had an ablation which served me very well.

However, I have noticed the inflammation (which I think is related to the mesh tape) is worse at menstruation! I am nearly 53, am not particularly physically fit and a little over weight (I weigh 12.5 stone and am 5.5 feet tall!).

I will be recovering from the trials of having the mesh removed and also the hysterectomy. I swing from minute to minute; to just have one operation done and then go back for the other one if I am still in pain? Or have it all done together and have one massive healing.

My consultant thinks she can remove the womb through the vagina however as it is palpable although large, if not she will have to intervene with abdominal surgery.

I have so many concerns, recovery time, downtime, back to work, pain levels, will I be more at risk of pelvic organ prolapse, will sex be the same or will there be no feeling left afterwards, as the womb plays a part in sex and contractions.

The Start Of My Journey, Sharyn Butler

I am now 63 years old. I have three daughters, all natural births. My husband and I were publicans and had a very busy life with the pub and also doing catering and running a bed and breakfast. I enjoy retirement but missed the contact with people that I had in my busy life.

I decided to join a couple of keep fit classes, one of them was Jazzasize and I loved it! It's then I believe that the prolapse started and it showed its ugly face (excuse the pun).

After months of putting up with the symptoms which the only way I could describe was I felt like I was turning into a man! It may sound funny but it wasn't very nice.

For the last few months it had ruled my life and when I was told I needed a full hysterectomy I was worried but relieved. I had finally realized it was quite common and it would help me.

I had my operation three days ago and hopefully my journey back to normality begins now.

Hoping For A Silver Lining, Amanda

I have finally been given the chance to have a hysterectomy after around 10 years of symptoms!!

I didn't know what the problem was at first, I just kept getting exhaustion and anaemia. I have had two large babies (16 and 21 years old now) by c-section and increasingly, over the last five years in particular, I have been suffering with lower back pain, swelling of the abdomen and pain in one hip and down the leg and utter, utter exhaustion. It never occurred to me that the hip pain would be connected to my uterus! I was sent for a scan of my hip, which came back normal. I then had a Mirena coil fitted for four years, which stopped my periods completely and was great while it lasted but the hip pain never went away and was, in fact getting worse. Eventually I had it removed (the Mirena, not the hip!)

Last autumn I started having heavy bleeds. These were not heavy periods, I knew that, but kept being told they were just heavy periods. We know our own bodies. Apart from the fact that they were not in any pattern, the blood flow was too red and far too clotty and the flow was relentless. During the worst bleed I ended up in my doctor's surgery where she took one look at the state I was in and told me to go straight to A&E. Luckily enough I did not need a transfusion and eventually the bleeding stopped. To date I have had four of these bleeds. One in October, two in January four days apart and one in March.

After a further scan by a specialist it was discovered that the large fibroid I'd been told I had for many years was actually a focus of adenomyosis (or a large adenomyoma). My uterus was bulky and I had adenomyosis in all of it. From what I have been told I had been having some kind of rupture and this is what was bleeding.

I have never ever felt so tired in all of my life. I can honestly say that it is debilitating as some days I cannot get out of bed and on others I have to have an afternoon sleep; not good when you have a job. I find it so hard. My DH calls me Womble, as I am always tidying up and organising stuff but at the moment I cannot operate normally at all.

I am scheduled to have a hysterectomy in two weeks and I cannot wait to have my uterus taken away. Fingers crossed that I will start feeling better again after 10 years of living with it.

Recognising Endometriosis And Adenomyosis, Elaine

I feel so very sad reading all the comments posted on the website. So many women face such a dreadful decision and most of them after having already put up with years of misery.

I have had menstrual problems for ages. I had heavy and painful, irregular periods in my teens, and was put on the pill. Not that the pill did any good, it just gave me spots, bloating and mood swings. I gave that up pretty quickly and just decided to put up with my menstrual pain. This settled down for a little while during my 20s, and I successfully completed university, began my career, and met a great guy.

My problems started again in agonising earnest in 2002. I had very heavy and painful periods, which could be anything between three and six weeks apart. I bled for anything up to 9-10 days. My periods were generally full of clots, and I suffered dreadful pains and cramping. I have suffered anaemia constantly as a result, and have tried all sorts of iron supplements, including Ferrograd, Ferrous Fumarate, Ferrous Sulphate, Sanatogen, Minadex, vitamins with iron but nothing works. They just upset my stomach really badly.

Over the years, I've felt steadily worse – really run down. I am constantly terribly fatigued, and have almost permanent lower back pain (worse on the right). I also get terrible cramps and pelvic pain in the lead up to my period, as well as water retention and bloating (I can gain up to seven pounds in less than a week). I do not feel in control of my body, my moods or hormones, and this makes me feel stressed, and drained. I have breakouts of spots, and am constantly tired and achy. It's like living permanently with the symptoms of flu. I also get night sweats and hot flushes. This can be extremely embarrassing, as I sweat terribly, but I have no idea what suddenly brings the hot flushes on.

I am now only 41, so this cannot be the menopause. My symptoms are so debilitating, there are days I could just sit and cry. I feel so very angry that so little is being done to help me. I live with constant pain and fatigue. I am also extremely vulnerable to infections – I get multiple respiratory infections every year, as well as thrush, and urinary infections. It's reached a point where my GP (who is desperately insensitive) just fobs me off with antibiotics over the telephone!

I've been going to the GP about this for years, with no support whatsoever. I was initially given numerous misdiagnoses, including irritable bowel, stress and food intolerances. I was referred to a gynaecologist in 2006, and he misdiagnosed polycystic ovaries. Following this, I was told again to try the Pill – Dianette and then Marvelon (neither of which worked).

In 2008, I had a hysteroscopy with D&C. Afterwards; my gynaecologist told me he found 'no reason for my symptoms'. This is despite the fact that the locum I saw for my hysteroscopy (because my usual gynae was off sick) recorded endometriosis and possible adenomyosis in my notes! I also got referred for a colonoscopy, due to dreadful bowel symptoms of diarrhoea and bloating, and the bowel surgeon again suggested endometriosis. My gynaecologist completely overlooked this, as did my GP (who is useless). Instead, I was told to try the Mirena device. Again, this had NO effect at all. I still got pain, and flooding with every period. It was a nightmare at work, and my employers (I was a social worker) were utterly unsupportive. I just got treated like a malingerer who made a fuss over simple period pain!

In the meantime, I had to argue with my GP as I wanted a second opinion, which they were refusing. I was made to feel a right nuisance! I was even told to take Prozac, as my GP tried to convince me I was 'clinically depressed'. I'll admit, by this time (2008) I probably was beginning to feel pretty low. Quite simply, I had been ignored and made to feel like a fusspot for years. Nobody seemed to take my pain and other symptoms seriously.

In late 2009, I was pushed out of my job. I'd got utterly sick by this point of all the nastiness and lack of sympathy at work. I was constantly being reprimanded for having to have time off and attending medical appointments. Every period was dreadful – my symptoms were such a nuisance at work, but I was made to feel I had to soldier on.

In 2010, my husband complained to the GP as by now I was constantly anaemic, with very heavy and painful periods, and chronic back pain. My career and social life were dead, and my sex life non-existent due to pelvic pain. I finally got a second opinion in late 2010, and was instantly told I had endometriosis and needed urgent surgery. I was gobsmacked! Like, how did they suddenly know so quickly?

I've since had three surgeries, and several hospitalisations. April 2011 – laparoscopy and laser ablation. May 2011 – hospitalised due to pain. July 2011 – A&E due to crippling back pain. August 2011 – ambulance emergency, taken to hospital, and hospitalised due to crippling pain in back and pelvis. Adhesions suspected. Physiotherapy assessment, and discharged with crutches, which I needed for nearly three weeks. December 2011 – more ablation and also a radical check of my pelvic cavity to look for more endometriosis, which was found as nodules deep inside my uterosacral ligaments. Adhesions and surgical scarring were also found. March 2012 – another laparoscopy, with laser ablation and radical surgical resection of my scarring, adhesions and excision of endometriosis from my uterosacral ligaments.

I have no children, and am 41. I lost a baby due to miscarriage in early 1994. Late 1994, I was pregnant again, but ended up having a termination, as my ex-boyfriend decided he did not want to be a dad. I was easily coerced into having the termination, as I began to bleed again during the pregnancy, and was terrified I'd miscarry again.

Talking recently to my mum, she tells me of a family history of miscarriage and menstrual problems. Mum miscarried once before having me, and also had period problems. Her sister had a hysterectomy for fibroids and other associated period problems. My Nan had anaemia and menstrual problems. I have a cousin with endometriosis and breast cancer, and a further aunt who died of ovarian cancer.

I am in constant pain, and rarely get a week every month that is free of symptoms. These include bloating, upset stomach, nausea, water retention, chronic pain, fatigue, cramping, and heavy, irregular periods. It's been confirmed that I have endometriosis, and my gynae says it's probable I have adenomyosis as well. I also have anaemia, asthma, chronic sinusitis and M.E. No treatment so far has worked.

I am desperate and considering hysterectomy as a last option. I am so scared and upset. I have no idea what to do for the best. I cannot stand my symptoms anymore; they have ruined my life. But I am also scared of what I may feel once I have lost my final chance to have children. I already feel a failure as a woman.

Be Prepared, Diane Leakey

Hopefully my story is an empowering one as there is so much negativity around this subject and my experience wasn't.

My experience around the whole thing has been very positive but then I did invest a lot of time and effort before the operation and that is my BIG TOP TIP. Prepare both physically and mentally beforehand.

Get as fit as you can before the event, invest in some excellent shoes for walking after the operation and get your friends motivated to take you out walking. I was up walking outside the hospital by day three and walking 30 minutes by day five. But then I did lots of gentle jogging and some weight training before that helped. I therefore didn't get depressed I just went for a walk. By the end of six weeks I was walking three hours! Everyone gave me great encouragement to get walking, especially the nurses on the ward.

Get your mind around if you want any hormone replacement treatment, and if so what, again before the event. I decided on patches and was adamant I wanted them the day after the operation. They worked and I've felt fine since, although the dose did need to be raised.

I stocked up on DVDs to watch, books to read and projects to do. In the end I had too many but that's better than being bored.

Bending is a problem so get a table next to where you intend to base yourself during the day – it's for your stuff and absolutely no one, under pain of death, can put any of their trash on it.

The golden rules when you come home are REST, WATER and EXERCISE. Do this religiously, you can't drink enough water, I've covered the exercise bit and as for the rest just don't feel guilty. See it as a present for you to do your stuff you'll never get this luxury again.

Reflecting back, six months after my total abdominal hysterectomy for fibroids (two grapefruit size with numerous smaller ones) I don't have any gripes, everyone was fantastic and very supportive. However I was amazed at how tired I felt. Be kind on yourself and don't expect to be fully back to normal at six weeks. I'm still amazed how tired I still feel.

A Man's Best Friend Is His Wife, Roger

I came across the website whilst Googling for information to help me understand just what my wife would be going through both operatively and post-operatively. I must say I have found it extremely informative and helpful, I would definitely urge anyone who needs good advice and information to visit and sign up for the weekly hints and tips.

From my point of view, as a mere male, I would advise all men whose wife / partner is having to contemplate a hysterectomy for whatever reason to do a few things.

Firstly, take the trouble to understand the female anatomy, this is most important.

Secondly go with their partner to all appointments from the initial consultation onwards.

Do go to the hospital with her to give support and re-assurance on the day of the operation. Go with her to the entrance to the operating theatre and then wait so that you can be there when she awakes and returns to the ward afterwards.

Read all of the information that the hospital will supply and definitely visit the Hysterectomy Association website where even more advice can be found.

At all times be prepared to talk to your partner about how she feels, what exactly she is having done and how you can help. But most importantly always re-assure her that it will in no way change the way you feel about her.

My wife is still a woman and still the woman I love and will always remain so, and I am glad to say that she knows this because I have told her so. I have been fortunate in having the time to spend making sure that life at home has been restful for her and have seen the benefits of ensuring that she has not done anything that she was advised not to do.

I accompany her on a short walk each day and take each day as it comes.

I appreciate that this may seem strange coming as it does from a man, but I think that there ought to be booklets aimed at us so that we can help our partners by being armed with the correct and sensible knowledge from the start, and that they should be given out by the hospital staff at the first consultation.

Very many thanks for the support the site has enabled me to give to my very precious wife.

Before, Yvonne

The roar of the traffic was like the wind whispering through trees compared to the blood pulsing through my ears. I remember the deep gulps as I steadied myself against a railing outside of the hospital and rang my husband.

My consultant, one of the top three consultants in the UK for hormonal problems, had shaken his head gently. There were no more options. My problem, he'd explained, is that I simply can not tolerate progesterone. Not the progesterone my own body makes, nor an artificial version. And, he said, if you have a uterus, you have to have the progesterone.

Surely I can take a smaller dose, I'd said. I was crying, but it was nothing to do with the conversation content. My PMS had been chronic for nearly eight years, and I was utterly, utterly drained that day. I'd had several weeks of dropping asleep in the most inappropriate places (including on the loo in work, with my head resting against the toilet roll holder), and I was physically in a great deal of pain. Trying to listen, and comprehend his words with my muffled hearing was difficult. But it was a difficult message to receive too.

He said, you already take a dangerously low level and look at you. You can't cope with it. I wanted to reassure him, tell him that it would pass, but in my heart I knew that I'd reached the end of the line.

Okay, I'd said. Pulling my coat on, I'd just nodded when he told me to book in the operation as soon as possible, and he reiterated that I needed everything removed. He said some long words about the name of the operation. I've never repeated them; I've never paid any heed to the actual detail of the operation nor the scarring. Right then, I just knew I needed to talk to my husband and get him to talk to the insurance company.

My hands shook as I was calling, grateful to my core once again that my husband's job came with private medical insurance. I'd certainly taken full advantage of it when, just a year ago, I decided that I needed to take control and find a solution, wherever that solution led me. I couldn't cope.

There was a long silence after I'd told my husband what had happened while the words hung on the line between us. We'd both known, really, that we'd done as much as we could. Science had no more remedies for us to try, and I think part of us both felt a sort of relief.

Can it wait, he'd asked, until after our holiday in September? It was June. I wanted to say no, but it wasn't just me that was affected, was it. (to be continued .....)

DURING

It's 3am, Day Five Post-Op, Annie Martyn

I had my operation five days ago. I am writing this at 3am whilst contemplating whether I should try going to the toilet – a frightening prospect but reading this I no longer feel alone. I don't have the pain many seem to have (except for poo and wind pain) and I've not needed the pain killers given by the hospital, although this in itself worries me – do anti-inflammatory have other benefits (i.e. reduce the swelling) as well as pain relief?

I'm very fit; three days before my operation I was climbing the highest mountain in North Africa's Atlas Mountains but now I'm going crazy being able to do so little. I'm allowing myself a few days of comfort eating but am terrified of weight gain – I used to be morbidly obese so I'm going to have to keep that in check.

This is less of a story and more of a thank you. At 3am sometimes you just need to tell someone how you feel. Right toilet beckons – wish me luck!

Update: three months on I was able to run 6k comfortably and today I'm weight training three times a week as I'm booked to do a rescue diving course requiring me to be able to lift a man from the ocean. The weight did go on but it's gone again quickly and I've never felt healthier. The hysterectomy for me was definitely the best thing I could have done!

21 Days Post-Op And No Pain, Samantha Balfre

Hi ladies, I thought I would share my story as I feel I am extremely lucky and for those of you who are worrying just like I was it's not always pain and more pain. Unlike many ladies my journey to my hysterectomy was a bit of a whirlwind and I did not have to go through years of suffering and waiting.

I am 46 and thought everything was fine until July 2012, when I was rushed into hospital with really heavy bleeding. I was kept in overnight and after having a scan was told that I had fibroids and a bulky uterus which at the time I didn't know what they meant.

I was sent home with Tranexamic acid tablets which I was told to take as soon as my period started to help control the bleeding. These worked great and in fact stopped the bleeding within a day. Then in October I went to the toilet one morning and found I had this large lump poking out of me, thought I was turning into a lady boy and was scared stiff.

I went to the doctors where my worries weren't helped when she said she had never seen anything like it. So off to the hospital I went, where the consultant told me it was a fibroid on a stalk that had prolapsed through my cervix. He said it was approximately 8cm long and 6cm in diameter. When I got to the hospital it had gone back inside me slightly, the consultant said that my uterus was also the size of someone 22 weeks pregnant and that the best thing, having also looked at my previous scan results, would be to have a total abdominal hysterectomy.

Slightly shell-shocked I was sent home with some new tablets that had just finished their trials called Esmya which I was told should stop the bleeding altogether which they did and start shrinking the fibroids. My date came through a couple of weeks later for 13th December 2012.

I started looking online for information and speaking to friends who had also had hysterectomies. I found the HA which is amazing and so helpful; but the more I read and was told, the more scared I became about the amount of pain I would be in. I am on my own so didn't have anyone to share my fears with.

Thursday 13th December came and I trundled off to hospital. I met with the consultant again who went through the operation; after reading and speaking to others I had decided to keep my ovaries. I then saw the anaesthetist who told me he would give me a spinal tap before the anaesthetic to put me to sleep for the op.

When I woke up in recovery, I was in some pain but nowhere near as much as I was expecting. I had a catheter and drip but no drain and I also wasn't on patient controlled analgesia which I was expecting. The oxygen made me cough constantly and because of this I drank loads; the nurses were quiet shocked how much I was drinking. I had to stay in recovery for three hours as there no beds on the ward and just before I went up I was giving some oral morphine.

Once on the ward, apart from the constant checks from the nurses, I slept. I was given painkillers as prescribed but was still quite numb from the spinal tap and to be honest was dreading when that wore off. The next morning the doctor came and saw me, he said they had to remove my left ovary due to there being a cyst but that everything else had gone okay.

The catheter was removed and I was taken off the drip, the spinal tap had worn off and surprisingly I was still in hardly any pain. The nurses got me up and after going to the bathroom I went off for a little walk. The nurses again were shocked at how good I was and how I was walking completely upright, although a bit slowly, as if nothing had happened. This surprised me as well, I'm not the fittest of people and everyone had said how the pain was so bad that they walked hunched over.

Friday was spent mostly dozing again with pain killers given only at prescribed times. Saturday morning came and I was told I could go home; then the dreaded trapped wind got me. I can honestly say I have never been in so much pain in all my life so going home was put off. Although the first nurse I kept speaking to did nothing, just leaving me there for hours doubled up in agony; when another nurse found me in pain she immediately gave me a gynae cocktail, which is warm water, peppermint and other things, within 15 minutes the wind was flowing from both ends and the pain finally went away.

By Sunday I was three days post-op and went home; the only pain killers I was on were paracetamol and ibuprofen. Apart from the strange grumblings and feelings inside my stomach, which I still get occasionally now, there was hardly any pain; in fact by the end of the second week post-op I was off the pain killers altogether.

Sleeping is a bit hard; I usually sleep part on my side and part on my belly. I tried sleeping on my back and I now wedge a pillow under both sides of me, so if I do turn on my side my belly is supported. My scar started weeping in a couple of places but I have been to the doctors who swabbed it and dressed it and have confirmed there is no infection. Apart from that everything is going remarkably well.

I only had slight bleeding after the op and this stopped by the Saturday. I have not been tired or weepy. My biggest problem now, because I am not in pain, is remembering I have had major surgery and not to do too much. I have a friend who walks my dog for me and a couple of others pop in and out and do stuff for me. Being on my own I am used to doing everything and I have to stop myself.

I do have a swollen belly and am living in my pj's as that's about all I can get on. I find if I do too much my belly goes numb (a bit like when you've been for a filling) and swells even more, but I feel so very lucky not to be in pain.

I would just like to say to all you ladies out there waiting for your ops, good luck and it's not always painful and my advice is to take arnica, I did and had hardly any bruising. If the oxygen mask makes you cough ask for the one that goes in your nose rather than the mask over your mouth; it tickles to start with but is so much better than the mask, and makes drinking etc. so much easier. Drink loads of water and if you have trapped wind ask for a gynae cocktail; it doesn't taste nice but works wonders.

Be prepared for the first time you move your bowels afterwards, I was in the toilet for ages once I started. If you are in pain take everything you are offered, if not in pain remember what you have had done. Invest in big knickers, either from the Hysterectomy Association site or I bought maternity support knickers and they really do help, and lastly I hope you all have a speedy and good recovery. X

From A Healthy Life To Total Abdominal Hysterectomy In 3 Months, Carol

I was fine until a week after my 47th birthday when I was admitted to hospital with gall stones. An ultrasound and laparoscopic operation removed the gall stones but the radiographer reported an ovarian cyst to investigate later. GP checked my CA125 as a routine – it was over 800! An ultrasound and MRI scan meant I ended up on January 30th having a TAH with both ovaries out. I am now waiting for the test results.

It's all such a shock. My husband, a total rock, is equally worried. The operation went fine, now sore and bored. The ladies on the website are a great support but I feel like the only one not to suffer symptoms. If it's your turn soon go for it, stay strong!

Recovery, Marie

Haven't really had chance to mull over what's happened as things happened so fast. I had a routine colonoscopy in February and the consultant felt a fibroid so suggested a gynae scan. The colonoscopy came back all clear and my symptoms were put down to IBS.

The gynae scan also told me everything ok but they insisted I saw a doctor. The blood test showed inflammation of my ovaries and within a week I saw another consultant. They suggested an MRI scan, which I had following day and a CT scan the following week.

I then went on holiday for three weeks. I came back to an appointment where the outcome showed a strange looking fibroid and it was suggested I have a complete hysterectomy; removing my womb, ovaries and lymph nodes as they were swollen and fibroid.

A week later on 24th April I was in.

I was out of it the first night but after a wash the next day I was sitting in a chair. My catheter was removed that night so of course I was getting up and down all night. The following day was more sitting and resting plus lots of trapped wind discomfort.

I was allowed home on the Saturday with stockings and anti thrombosis injections. I was glad to be home but felt every pothole on the drive back! It was lovely to get into my own bed but the difficulty was getting out. I tried a rope contraption so I could pull myself up but it was only half successful.

The next day I felt wonderful. I pottered around, watched some telly, the pain was ok and I thought this won't be so bad. But then I had a bad night as I was too warm, had restless legs and couldn't get comfy.

Consequently I didn't feel quite so perky the next day and this time I was on my own.

I managed okay though and pottered around again doing some needle felting. I had a fantastic 3rd night as I managed to lie on my side but today six days after op I feel really tired.

I think I did too much on Sunday but hopefully things will improve. I just have to wait for the appointment to discuss the biopsy results now.

I Will Feel 17 Again, Paula

I am now day nine post total abdominal hysterectomy to remove fibroids. I'm 45 years old, and hadn't expected anything like this to happen to me. I'd never really had any major gynae problems, and I'm not one to go to the doctors unnecessarily, so it all came as a bit of a surprise.

However, over recent years I'd felt like I had something heavy inside me that was like being pregnant. I was beginning to worry and I was getting pains and pressure on my other organs so decided to go to my GP. I'd first thought I may have problems with my ovaries, so my GP referred me for a scan.

Luckily I have private medical insurance through work, and was able to contact a very good gynaecologist a number of friends had recommended. She examined me and straight away knew from the large lump in my tummy that I had fibroids. She recommended further investigation which involved a laparoscopy under a general anaesthetic. I was surprised that even this op meant I felt unable to return to work for two weeks post op.

Between me and the consultant we decided to leave it a few months to see how I coped. At 45 and heading towards menopause the thought was that my fibroids would eventually shrink. We did discuss the Mirena coil, but I'd heard a few nightmarish stories from friends, and decided if I could live with out it then great.

I actually left it a whole year. I had good months but when I look back the bad months far outweighed the good ones. I felt that although I'd joined a gym and wanted to get fit, I was struggling with the pressure on my tummy. I was getting increased bloating and pain in my back. I was also struggling with indigestion and felt like I was seven months pregnant.

In February I went back to see my consultant. When she examined me she immediately felt that the largest of my fibroids had grown. She looked at me and asked me how I'd feel about a hysterectomy. I had expected as much and knew from our last meeting that it might be on the cards.

Luckily for me I have a very supportive husband and work for a large employer so the recovery time was not an issue. A part of me did think! OMG, I am now officially old! In my head I am still 17! However, I knew it was for the best and that I'd never feel totally well until I got it sorted out.

As I didn't have any ovarian problems I was able to keep my ovaries and tubes, but we decided to remove my cervix as I'd had a loop cone procedure in my 20's to treat CIN3 pre cancerous cells.

I was going to have the operation privately which meant I was able to chose a date to coincide with a less busy period at work. I also ensured it was after my birthday!

The operation went well, even though my consultant said it was a very difficult op. A lot of the fibroids were attached to various bits of my insides. I was offered an epidural along with my general anaesthetic, and as I'd had one before during childbirth (c-section), I accepted. Although I'd not remembered how uncomfortable it was! I assume the pain of childbirth meant the epidural was a walk in the park! It did help the post op pain and I was also given fluids and antibiotics through a drip as well as Paracetamol! I was surprised that Paracetamol was so effective intravenously!

I was in hospital for five days (four nights). Initially I struggled with pain the first day. The hospital had also given me Oxycontin, which is a 12 hour pain relief tablet. It's a strong barbiturate so I wasn't keen to keep this going although it did work very well! However, for the first few days I took some co-codamol which helped. The biggest issue for me was constipation! I didn't go for five days which was excrucia ting. However, I increased my fibre intake, taken some gentle laxatives and it seems to be improving.

On day nine I am still very sore, and finding it hard to go the whole day without sleeping. However, I am moving about much more, and am taking it easy. I do feel guilty watching my husband run around like a headless chicken all the time just getting up from my dinner and sitting in front of the TV. I feel like I'm being lazy! He's back to work tomorrow and my parents are coming to pick me up so I can spend the day with them. I am hoping that in 6-8 weeks time I will feel like the 17 year old again!

I'd Never Had A Major Op Before, Carol Mcleod

Yes I was scared, really frightened about the 'what if's' – nobody and nothing prepares you for that walk to the theatre and knowing that when you come out – you are coming back – you'll be as helpless as a kitten and wired on pain relief. 12:10pm when they knocked me out, I remember the clock on the wall in room outside theatre, a quick glance as the orderly promised me a G&T when it was all over.

3:30pm when I woke up – freezing cold and shivering. Apparently that's the anaesthetic working its way out of the body system. Remembering my pre-op meeting with the nurse about a week before the op she'd told me if I was cold it was likely they'd given me an epidural and told me to wiggle my toes and fingers to get the blood moving. My toes feel distant, but coming back to me. Continuing my own system check I seem to be all still there! I'm trying to recall the chat I had with the nurse about a week before the op, she'd checked my blood, general health and talked me through what to expect before and after the operation. She'd offered advice on preparing for the operation, all of which turned out to be very useful.

More wiggling and the feelings are coming back, noticeably no pain. Deep breaths, the oxygen mask is there and will stay on for a couple of hours, a few deep breathes helps move the anaesthetic out of the system and helps healing. The pain control device in the back of my hand and is slightly skewed. It hurts when I move my hand. I've given the morphine a test blip as requested and float off – don't suffer pain, it's there to help with recovery. Thankfully I don't need it much over the next 18 hours and it's removed the following morning. My mouth and throat are painful – ventilation during the op I'm told. It's like having tonsillitis – a good excuse for a nice sweetie now and again.

Back on the ward I'm so hungry! At first I wasn't sure I'd cope with food but I can honestly say that's close to the best chicken sandwich and cup of coffee I ever had. The day before the op I'd eaten lots of fruit and drunk lots of water. The nurse had offered me that advice too for getting the digestive system functioning normally again after the op. Keeping on drinking after getting back to the ward was important too, it restores the hydration lost during the op and with systems working normally it's one step closer to getting out of hospital. It worked for me.

The amount of bleeding I hadn't prepared for, it continued through the night but didn't cause the nurses any concern. By the time the packing and catheter were removed in the morning it had stopped completely. That allowed me freedom again – shower, slow walks along the corridor and three days after getting to the hospital I was home. There were a couple of difficult days about a week after the op.

My whole system seemed to have some sort of shut down – a delayed shock perhaps. I knew I had done the right thing, all had gone according to plan, and the surgical team were happy. Now mind and body just needed to heal. Yes it takes time and I did come through. The physical wounds heal – I'm still amazed I was glued back together and have no scars at all. I couldn't help but check morning and night it was still holding together – although I've no idea what I would have done if it had broke! Mentally I'm not one to dwell on stuff – I had little choice in having this op so I tried to stay optimistic and positive and get through it. It's a few years on now, I don't regret or question the decision and I still feel the better for it.

There were four of us in the ward having the same op. For some the trauma of it all was clear on their face. What's also clear is that it is different for everyone so knowing as much as you can and being clear about it before the op helps so much afterwards. That said I think I would still be that frightened all over again. And the orderly still owes me the G&T!

Life Altering Surgery For Some, Carole C. O'Brien

I had my hysterectomy on February 13th of this year. The procedure was done robotically, by the da Vinci method. This meant my body was slanted almost straight up and down and a complete hysterectomy was done. The da Vinci robot magnifies everything inside 10-12 times so it is easier for the surgeon to see and to make sure he/she doesn't nick or cut things other than what is to be removed. In my hysterectomy everything was removed, uterus, cervix, ovaries, fallopian tubes, etc. Thankfully, no cancer was found as the doctors I had seen (and I!) were concerned there would be.

I am at the 6th week in recovery today, Monday, March 26th. Tomorrow, March 27th I go back to the gynaecologist/oncologist surgeon to see if my internal sutures are healing as they need to.

My hysterectomy was done to see if there was cancer and if there was none, to prevent cancer, as I had to have a D&C and Hysteroscopy November 2009 and January 2010, respectively, due to bleeding after menopause. The bleeding had begun again this past November 2011 and was heavier and was still continuing each month including February just before my surgery.

The surgery was a three hour operation and I have five incisions in my abdomen, the largest one being above my naval, but all have healed well. I have had lots of fears and apprehensions, beginning while in the hospital with my bladder not working on its own and needing to come home with a catheter. Thankfully, the catheter was able to be removed five days later and my bladder has been working fine on its own since then!

The website has been the greatest help to me that I have been able to find as my surgeon did not have any printed information for me prior to or after the surgery (I did not think to ask for any prior to the surgery. I was so afraid of cancer I could not think of anything besides making sure whether or not I had it and if not, preventing it) and the hospital did not have any printed information for me either. When I asked for printed information after my surgery from the gynaecologist/oncologist, his reply was that his office doesn't give out information because most people wouldn't understand it anyway. If I had been told that prior to the surgery, I have a feeling I very probably would have looked for yet another gynaecologist and gotten another opinion.

As a 68 year old mother of six now-grown children, who was a farm wife while raising my children, being told after my surgery at the time of my dismissal from the hospital 'do not lift for two weeks' and then on the day the catheter was removed that I was to 'do nothing for six to eight weeks,' but having no other instructions left me in the dark information-wise much more than I realised and phone calls to the surgeon's nurse and the hospital did not result in being given any printed information. In fact they each gave me information that was very different from what the doctor had told my husband and me. The instructions from the surgeon's nurse and from the nurse on the surgical floor at the hospital when I called those places a few weeks after my surgery to try to find information to help me was very depressing as well as disturbing because their instructions were so different from the surgeon's.

The forums and other information on the website have been and are a godsend to me. I know I will continue looking through the website and gathering information from other women's experiences that will help me to continue to know I am not alone and I will make it through this safer than I might have otherwise.

My bowels are still a concern to me, as in order to not have a painful movement and to get the movement started I have to raise my shoulders up toward my ears, pulling my body as upright as possible. Also, because of having an operation on the sphincter muscle in my rectum, it is necessary almost daily to put toilet tissue on my hand and push on the right outside area of my rectum. I can feel the bowel movement sitting there and as I push I am able to get the bowel movement started and then my body continues to relieve itself on its own. I am hoping this will not be a permanent situation or at least the fear of the pain if I strain will soon be gone. I can deal with the rest, as I have had that problem off and on since having the rectal surgery in 1993.

Drinking prune juice or eating prunes is very helpful, but it is hard to find the 'happy medium' or 'right balance' and not end up with having my stools too loose and then having my sphincter muscle unable to hold and I don't want to have an accident in my underwear!

If I could have done anything different, it would have been what I am doing now, as a much too late afterthought. but if I had known about it before having a hysterectomy, it might possibly have helped me to avoid having to have a hysterectomy, but none of the doctors I went to ever mentioned it and I didn't have the knowledge then that I have now. I have had my hormone levels tested and I am currently using bio identical hormones to try to get my hormones balanced, as they (and I!) have been a mess for several months. I wish so much that someone would have tested my hormones before telling me I HAD to have a hysterectomy and worked with hormones to see if my problems would straighten out instead of having to have the hysterectomy.

Three doctors, one a female family practitioner, another who was a male OBGYN and the third one, a male oncologist/gynaecologist, all told me I HAD to have a hysterectomy because otherwise I was going to have cancer. None of them ever mentioned possible hormone problems and/or addressing them if they were there, and then at my final post-surgery doctor appointment I was told that even though a woman's ovaries have been removed, it is still possible for her to get ovarian cancer.

That was and still is very shocking information. Words of caution from me to any woman who is told she MUST have a hysterectomy would be to find every bit of information you can about your situation before having a hysterectomy. When you have done that, you won't be left as I have been with always wondering if the hysterectomy could have been prevented.

I have struggled with depression and anxiety for most of my life and being able to have an orgasm always helped me to relax and was a very important part of my life. Since the hysterectomy that part of my life is nearly non-existent except on very rare occasions, for which I am very thankful. I am hoping and praying that as I continue with the bio identical hormone treatments, I will do better in that part of my life. I am very thankful to have a very understanding husband who has gone with me to each of my appointments and who sincerely cares about my well being and our life together – not just his own personal needs.

My words of advice would be that if it is not an imperative that a hysterectomy is done immediately, that each one of you would check out every option before going through a hysterectomy that might possibly be able to be avoided.

Being able to find the Hysterectomy Association has been my saving grace and I will be forever thankful.

A hysterectomy is a much more life altering surgery for some of us than for others, especially someone who has problems with depression and anxiety as I have had all of my life. I forgot to enter in my story that just before I went to the gynaecologist/oncologist who did my surgery, I had an appointment with the OBGYN that was supposed to be for a consultation only.

However, while in the middle of talking with my husband and me, he told us he had decided he was going to do a biopsy on me while I was there. What we didn't know and didn't ask him, was what kind of biopsy he was planning to do. After my husband left the room and the doctor left for me to get into a gown, the OBGYN came back in with a nurse and he did an endometrial biopsy, giving me nothing for the pain before, during or after.

The biopsy was a biopsy straight from hell and even though I have had six babies with nothing for pain, I cried out in pain as he cut into my body. The nurse came to my side and held me while he continued to cut on me. When he finished and left the room, the nurse made sure I was okay as I got dressed, but while doing that she told me that she was a surgical nurse and she was shocked, as she had never seen any doctor do to a patient what that doctor had done unless the patient was put to sleep first.

When the doctor came back into the room after I was dressed he told me to go to the appointment desk and schedule an appointment to be seen by him and another OBGYN the following week. In a state of shock, I did as he told me to and went home in pain and bleeding worse than I had before ever going to him. I called my family doctor and told her what had happened and she called my pharmacy and ordered a pill for me for pain. Needless to say, I cancelled the appointment I had scheduled while in shock and I have vowed to never, ever go to that doctor again and I can only hope and pray he does not do to others what he did to me.

I truly think I was still in somewhat of a state of shock when I went to the gynaecologist/oncologist who did my surgery, but since my family doctor had so much faith in him, even though the OBGYN had put me through hell, I was still too naive to ask questions that I now wish I had asked.

Not So Scary, Wendy

Hi, I've suffered with very heavy and painfully periods for years and years. I also suffered four miscarriages and two failed attempts at IUI. We are very lucky and very blessed to have eventually got pregnant and have a beautiful boy.

Four years after trying for another baba, with no results, continuous heavy bleeding with severe cramps and other problems, I demanded a full hysterectomy. I had tried all kinds of pills to stop bleeding, nothing worked.

After tests found out I had cysts and fibroids, I'd also had dodgy results in previous cervical smear tests so the surgeon suggested a total hysterectomy as my cervix was prolapsed. He also recommended a bladder repair as that had prolapsed too.

I could not wait to have my op as had suffered so much pain for so long, I was glad to get rid of everything. People kept saying to me you will go into the menopause straight away. But I'm not scared or worried about this; surely it can't be as bad as all the rubbish I have had to contend with for years.

I went into the hospital on the morning of the op, got a bit tearful as realisation and relief dawned on me; realisation that we would never get pregnant again and relief that it was all coming to an end.

Had my bloods, BP etc. done and then had to wait for three hours as the op wasn't booked until 2pm. I got gowned up and I was physically shaking by this time. Nurses put me to sleep (which is fab) and woke up, it seemed, minutes later. I was in quite a lot of pain and the nurse gave me morphine, which is also quite naughty but nice, she also put on an electric blanket as I was shaking.

I was taken back to my room and was very aware when my morphine wore off after every four hours, so buzzed for more. Have to say I didn't sleep too good that night as I had pads on my leg that kept expanding to keep my circulation going; also the nurse's were in and out to do my observations. I lay talking to one for ages. All the staff were amazing!

I had a bed bath the next morning and even went for a walk. I felt quite light headed but didn't pass out. I was attached to a catheter and had a drain from my tummy. I had no bleeding at all in my under wear, not even now 10 days later.

The WORST thing for me was taking out the vaginal pad! OMG! That was awful. And the trapped wind! I stayed in hospital for three and a half days.

I feel fab!

I just take pain killers (Paracetamol) when I need them. I feel some of the stories I was told before I went in were very dramatic. However, I was glad to get all my bits out and I do 'get on' with things so maybe my attitude helped.

Male Attitude To Female Patients, Name Withheld

I am a qualified medical scientist and lectured in pathology for 10 years. I thought I was prepared for my hysterectomy but, when I attended the pre-op appointment, I discovered that the estimated recovery period was six weeks for a TVH. As I had an interstate workshop (and needed to carry a 32kg case) within that time, I asked if there was a procedure which had a quicker recovery rate and was told that the Laparoscopically Assisted VH had a four week recovery.

I was given 24 hours to advise the hospital of my intention so went home and got on the Net to do some research. There was a dearth of information, but, as I could delay the op for six more weeks if I had the LAVH that's the one I opted for. However, it meant being operated on by someone other than my preferred surgeon.

A couple of days before the op, I discovered information relating to conserving the cervix and ovaries. I had already been told, at the pre-op consultation, that my ovaries would be spared but had been given no information on my cervix. I also had not been given a copy of my consent form. I called the patient advocate, at the (women's public) hospital and asked her to confirm with the surgeon that he would conserve my ovaries and cervix. I said I would not be proceeding unless he would. The response was that he would.

On the day of the operation, fasting, tired, apprehensive and five minutes before my operation I was told by the surgeon that he was not happy. He said that I might have endometrium in the cervix. So I agreed that it be removed. And asked if he was happy with that he said 'No, because your ovaries could be 'seeded' with tumour'.

I was in shock. I had understood that I had endometrial hyperplasia, with atypia, but no one had mentioned a risk of cancer. I asked if they could tell once they were inside the pelvis and he said 'No'. All I could think about was how many delays I had had before getting to this point (the hospital had mismanaged my hyperplasia and shunted me from clinic to clinic, for over a year, so that my condition had progressed to a more serious one). So I agreed for my ovaries to be removed.

Not only was the pathology of my ovaries normal, but I was told by the head of the unit that if I had had the TVH, my ovaries would have been spared. It was just that particular surgeon's preferred style!

Unfortunately, I had persistent pain and immobility (despite being extremely fit before the operation – gym four times a week) and it took me about 15 weeks to get back to work. The pain and discomfort had persisted for eight months, when the head of the unit examined me and found an extremely painful polyp (an aberration of the healing process) on my vaginal vault. He proceeded to remove it without telling me what he was doing and without an anaesthetic. Every fibre in my abdomen went into spasm and now six weeks later, I am still unable to have intercourse without a great deal of vaginal discomfort and abdominal pain.

Both the surgeons were male, one in his 30's and one in his late 50's and a former colleague of mine. I guess that they consider that a 58 year old woman does not need to have her sexuality or feelings taken into account when faced with an amputation of this magnitude and significance.

Some Stories Have Happy Endings, Caitlin

I am in my late 60s and have had a prolapse for four years. At first I had a pessary fitted which had to be changed and washed and then reinserted every six months. It worked perfectly at first but my consultant said at some stage, she'd have to perform a hysterectomy. I thought why, when the pessary worked so well. However, it began to cause problems recently as it rubbed against the womb causing a discharge. She said again that it was time for the op. but this fills me with fear. She said since I was past childbearing and I had children it was of no consequence. True, but I hate the thought.

I live on my own and fear I won't manage. One son lives a distance away and the other has a demanding partner. My girlfriends don't live near. I'm frightened of an infection. I'm frightened of the anaesthetic. I'm frightened of hospitals. My GP suggested I see a hypnotherapist. Has anyone else seen one for hospital phobias and can anyone suggest where to get help to overcome these fears. I realise I do have to have this op and I can't put it off forever.

Three months later and following one attack of shingles, one case of a urinary infection, and one cancellation, I finally had a vaginal hysterectomy. As the anaesthetist held the oxygen mask over my face and injected in my vein with the pre-med. I found myself thinking 'Death Row – here I come'. An hour and a half later I was back in my bed, alive and well but with a saline drip in one arm, a urinary catheter, and my legs wrapped with a pulsing compression bandage to stop embolism. I'd survived. I was discharged in three days, walking, talking and with such a sense of relief I felt like singing. The feelings of discomfort I'd lived with for so long had vanished. I was almost a new woman.

My advice is to gather as much information as you can or want to find out about your op. Make a list of questions to ask your consultant if possible or failing that, your GP. Don't be intimidated. Take a friend with you if you're scared. It's your body and you have a right to know and as I've just found out, some stories have a happy ending.

The Partner's Experience, Roseanna McCann

I am writing on behalf of my partner. We live in East Northamptonshire and the op was done at our local hospital.

It was decided in February 2012 that following an ultrasound and an internal investigation with a camera, that a full abdominal hysterectomy was required. The op was carried out mid September with admission into hospital for 7:30am on a Thursday morning. Op was from 11:30 till about 13:30 and then recovery. As is fairly usual a cut was made on the bikini line for about 6"- 8". She left hospital Sunday morning with, we were told no follow-up of any sort required.

As I write we have just been to a walk-in centre as one side of the scar is weeping and slightly infected – she is now on antibiotics.

Seven days after the operation she burst into uncontrollable tears, and we were told this is a combination of anaesthetic and hormones (her ovaries were left in place). She is feeling better each day and we hope the pain subsides once the infection is under control.

I Have A Lot To Look Forward To, Jackie Dainty

I had my surgery on 22nd November 2012, I had a 10cm growth on my right ovary which was a borderline tumour, I had a full abdominal hysterectomy, and also had my appendix removed. I am pleased to say that the histology came back clear, so it is onwards and upwards from here. I was cut from just above my belly button, right down to my nether regions, and had clips in which were removed after 10 days.

Post-op I had two pain bombs which were fed directly into the wound. I had my op first thing in the morning, and only got to the ward after 4pm as I apparently took a long time to come round, I was on oxygen overnight and IV pain relief. The biggest shock I had was being asked to get up the following day! It turned out to be easier than I thought, and the next day I got up by myself. My op was on the Thursday and I went home on the Sunday. As I already inject myself (I have arthritis and inject once a week to help with it) I took home a month's supply of blood thinning injections to do myself. This was my choice as they did offer to do them for me but I didn't see the point at the time as I am more than capable of doing them myself. With hind-sight that may have been the wrong decision only in that it would have given me some contact with a professional to speak to about the things that were happening to me during my recovery.

This is where the 101 book and website support became a lifeline, as I felt totally abandoned. My family were awesome and my mother-in-law spent every day with me the first week to help me, what I struggled with was whether what I was experiencing was 'normal' or something that I should speak to the doctor about (my doctor is fantastic but as with most GPs these days very difficult to get in to see as the surgery is so busy). I read your book in one sitting and it answered so many questions.

I am now six weeks down the line, and I go back to see my doctor in two days to see about the pros and cons of HRT and getting back to driving and work. My scar is still extremely uncomfortable and I am still in tracksuit pants, as I can't bear to have anything touching it, I am also still struggling with my bowels – horrific wind and pain when I finally go to the toilet, I am taking laxatives – the peppermint tea was a great hint and does help.

I was on Morphine before the op as I was in an extreme amount of pain and also had to slowly come off that, but it wasn't the ordeal that it was made out to be. I did it slowly and didn't suffer any untoward withdrawal symptoms (despite some members of my family being worried that I would be addicted to it); I am now down to take Co-codamol for pain relief.

If I were to advise anyone about how to tackle your post-op recovery I would say that it is a must to take it one day at a time and don't rush your recovery. I spent two days in a lot of pain due to trying to lift something that was way too heavy!

Sleep, I went from sleeping most of the day, to having afternoon sleeps, which progressed to naps and now although I am tired in the afternoon I don't feel the need to have a sleep. Get a copy of the '101 Handy Hints for a Happy Hysterectomy' it's brilliant!

I am extremely fortunate to have an understanding and supportive husband, which has made my recovery time so much easier – here is to 2013. I know I am getting better, and that I have a lot to look forward to now.

Emergency Hysterectomy After Having A Baby, Tasha

I was twenty four years old when I went into labour with my first child. My waters broke as soon as I woke up that morning, but after that labour was slow. After nearly 23 hours my doctor decided we should do a caesarean because the baby was stuck and wasn't descending through my pelvis the way she should. I was so exhausted that I agreed right away and they whisked me off to the operating room. Everything seemed to go fine, and after a few days in the hospital we were sent home.

Exactly 14 days later I bolted out of bed in the middle of the night, feeling like my waters had broken all over again. I rushed into the bathroom to find bright red blood filling my pad and underwear. I called out for my fiancé and told him to get my mother, who lives with us and is an emergency room nurse. She saw what was happening and quickly called an ambulance.

In the ER the doctor inspected me and I felt a gush of blood let loose from between my legs. The nurses were racing around trying to get blood from the blood bank but it was taking too long. The technician panicked and didn't understand their orders for O-, the universal donor blood. Finally they got me hooked up and pushed the cold fluids into my body. I was shaking uncontrollably from the chill.

My doctor showed up looking sad and scared. They called in a surgeon and I was taken into the operating theatre so they could put a medical balloon in my uterus in the hopes of stopping the bleeding for long enough to air lift me to a bigger hospital. They also wanted to do a D&C inspection to see if there was any placenta left in my uterus that might be causing the bleeding.

I awoke from the surgery and my doctor said that I was still bleeding and there wasn't time to take me to the city. They put me under again and cut along the barely healed c-section. When I woke up I no longer had a uterus, but the bleeding had finally stopped. I was in the ICU for a few days. I can hardly remember.

The pain was unbearable and I was constantly on the heaviest pain medications. The maternity nurses came in and helped me with a breast pump in the hopes that I could resume breastfeeding soon.

Once I was a bit more stable I was able to go back onto the maternity ward so that I could keep my two week old baby by my side. It was hard to believe that this little baby would be the only one I had, but I was still so grateful to have her and be alive.

Breastfeeding was a challenge after all my body had been through, but we kept up with it. I couldn't hold her in our normal cradle position because of the pain on my torso, so breastfeeding required lots of pillow arrangements and baby rearrangements. The nurses were very zealous in their support of breastfeeding, which was good because otherwise I would have given it up. My daughter had to be supplemented a few bottles of formula a day at first but slowly my milk came back and by the time she was three months old we were on all breast milk again.

It was really hard once I got back home (about a week later). I couldn't believe that I'd had a hysterectomy. I was overcome with grief at times. Holding a new born baby makes you think you could do it all again in a heartbeat, but that was never going to come again. I was still in a lot of pain.

Because the surgery was an emergency procedure they didn't have time to really make sure I would be comfortable. The skin around the surgery site was completely numb, though right where the numbness stopped there was a stabbing nerve pain. As I write this, six months on, my skin is still a little bit numb, but the pain is long gone.

In the first few weeks back at home I spent a lot of time looking at adoption agencies. It helped me to think that someday I could help out a little baby or child who needed a home. It took about a month before I could sleep next to my fiancé again. The surgery site hurt so badly that I was afraid to sleep next to him, for fear of him brushing against my stomach and accidentally causing me pain. It was good to be next to him again, it was a step towards our normal life again. The doctor okayed sex about eight weeks later, though it still took me some time before I was comfortable being intimate, it was even longer before I could truly let go of the fear.

I went to a counsellor a few times to help me let go of the anxiety that was constantly with me. It really helped to talk to someone about it, someone who was completely disconnected from my family and friends. Journaling my feelings helped me a lot too. I never held onto any anger at the doctors for what had happened, but the fear from coming so close to death still gripped me. Nightmares of it happening again plagued me, and I was left with a shadow of grief and fear. I was so grateful to be alive, yet a piece of me was gone.

Now, six months later, I feel normal again. Going for walks and getting strong helped me realize that I could depend upon my body. Journaling helped get the fears out of my head and onto paper, where it could be contained. I am so thankful to be alive and united with my beautiful little family.

I've Got My Life Back! Lita

I had my daughter by c-section in January 2000 and I never recovered my energy levels. It got so bad that I went to the doctor in summer 2001 and had a range of blood tests, none of which were out of the normal ranges. However I just got more and more tired and then in 2004, when I was swimming, I started getting cramping pains in my chest that lasted 24 hours. Again I went to the doctor and I was advised not to swim so hard. At Christmas 2006 I got a cough that I couldn't shift for months and still I was getting increasing tired and weaker. I stopped doing anything fun and just went to work and slept. In August 2007, while on a camping holiday, I got very bad cramping pains in my chest late at night that lasted about six hours. The following morning my ribs felt bruised and as soon as I started walking around, the cramping pains came back. I went to the on-site doctor, who listened to my chest and then made a phone call. He returned and said that he had spoken to A&E at the local hospital and they were expecting me.

In A&E an x-ray showed a shadow on my lungs but the doctors didn't know what it was. They decided to assume it was pneumonia and sent me away with strong antibiotics. Back home and two weeks later nothing had changed except that I was finding it increasing difficult to breathe. Another x-ray showed that the shadow was still there and I was referred to the respiratory section of my local hospital.

While waiting for an appointment, I collapsed several times and was admitted to hospital. I was in hospital for four weeks but despite numerous tests, including a PET scan, no diagnosis was reached. The chest pain by now was continuous and getting worse. Finally in February 2008 I was referred to the Royal Brompton Hospital and was operated on 16 days after my first appointment. The surgeon found cancer of the heart lining and had to remove part of the heart lining and half of my left lung. Luckily the cancer had spread out into my lung and not into my heart so the operation removed all the cancer and I didn't need either chemotherapy or radiotherapy. A week after the operation I was walking around and feeling better than I had for years.

However three weeks later I was back in hospital as an emergency with a pulmonary embolism. From then on I started going downhill, with difficult painful breathing, back pain, chronic fatigue, and dizziness and unable to walk more than a few steps without losing my balance. In autumn 2010 I started having difficulty urinating and defecating and was taught to self-catheterise and had to take large amounts of laxatives in order to move my bowels. My periods became increasingly heavy and I was bleeding most days. In September 2011 an ultrasound scan showed that my womb was much enlarged with multiple fibroids and that I had a large fibroid attached to the outside of my womb. My gynaecologist recommended a hysterectomy and in March 2012 I had an abdominal hysterectomy under epidural.

I'm now four weeks post surgery and I am a new woman. My breathing is normal, I can walk, the chronic fatigue has gone and so has most of the back pain. My bladder and bowels are improving daily and I hope that in time they will return to normal. I still tire quickly and have little stamina but I am now able to do 10 minutes aerobic exercise daily and I take a walk a couple of times a day. I've even started to do a little belly dancing using a DVD as suggested in 101 book. I wear a support girdle all day because I find this removes the dragging feeling that I get when I stand up for any length of time. (I tried the abdominal support band but it stops right on my scar.)

My hysterectomy was done to try to stop my general physical condition from deteriorating further but the weight and size of the fibroids both inside the womb and out were obviously the cause of all of my symptoms. I have gone from merely existing to living again. I am very grateful to live in a country where excellent medical services exist, even though it took nearly 11 years to get to the bottom of what was wrong with me. I know everyone is different but for me, my hysterectomy has been a life-saver!

On My Road to Recovery After My Hysterectomy, Chris S

Hi, I have just had my vaginal hysterectomy about two and a half weeks ago – not feeling too bad now. At the time I didn't know what to expect due to not reading the booklets and feeling sick looking at them.

I found the after-experience a worry with a lot of pains in my stomach and feeling tired. The thought of stretching and overdoing things while being on my own looking after five children, two of them teenagers who are not doing a lot.

I have no family, just a kind friend who has been a help and I've done pretty good. I did invest in a hand grabber which has helped a great deal in getting things I would not be able to achieve. I also had a bath seat and a mobility scooter to get around with.

I find now I am mobile enough to get around on my own without feeling tired which is a blessing in disguise. I hope my story is of help to you.

My Hysterectomy Story, Claire Edge

I found the website while researching my options a month ago and it certainly helped with my decision to have a hysterectomy. I had a failed ablation last November when my womb was perforated. Wish I'd had a plan B at the time and they'd done a hysterectomy there and then.

I had a total hysterectomy on 4th July and I was amazed at how little pain I had when I came round and for the first couple of days. I took everything possible after my ablation and was 'bunged up' for weeks (and thought I was going to die when I did eventually go!!). I was determined not to go through that again so went to hospital armed with peppermint cordial (very sweet and yucky), peppermint tea (brilliant and refreshing) and multivitamins with iron (as I'd had low levels a few week prior to the op)…and lastly, the attitude that I was going to be free of 'the curse'!!

One of the best pieces of advice I was given from a nurse was to put my feet on a box or step-stool, anything that would raise my knees when I went to the loo, it helped enormously.

The weirdest thing for me was my first ever experience of a catheter. I was fascinated and amazed by the amount of pee, 11 litres in 24hrs. I think it was a ward record! I was actually a bit sad when they took it out.

Staff in the hospital were amazing, they couldn't do enough for us and made us laugh, the best therapy of all. A physiotherapist came round every day to go through exercises to do immediately after the op and in the subsequent days/weeks and we were packed off with a booklet of the exercises. We were even asked what activities we wanted to get back to doing (such as dog-walking) and given realistic time-scales.

Naturally, being a woman who can't sit lounging around for too long, I did too much too soon and find myself in discomfort and a little emotional. Having just spoken to my consultant's assistant, I'm assured that what I'm feeling is perfectly normal and yes, I am doing too much!!

I actually find sitting and walking (i.e. going for a walk) the hardest things to do. Since my job involves sitting for most of the day, I'm not looking forward to the pain I know I'll encounter when I get home and relax. But I'll work on those supporting muscles, hopefully it will help.

Having seen some of the comments about lack of medical support, I can only say that while in hospital, I was given the best care I could have hoped for and a subsequent visit from the district nurse to remove my staples was equally brilliant. However, I know doctors and nurses are under immense stresses and, like most of us in these difficult times, are having to take on more responsibility and workload. So please don't be disheartened by the NHS, your GP or whoever – they may not have the resources to follow-up on every patient that comes through their door. If you are not recovering as well as you think you should be, or just want to speak to someone for reassurance, give them a call – I'm sure they will be more than willing and happy to help. OR…look through the fabulous website; it's packed with useful information and practical advice. Wishing you all a speedy and happy recovery. x

Horrible UTI, Dee Vadera

I guess I have been lucky on the whole compared to a lot of the stories I have read. I went in for a hysterectomy feeling confident that I was in good shape and everything would go according to plan. Well it did, except for one thing. I could not pass water when I was expected to. I tried every five minutes and was in agony as it was only the day after the operation. After seven hours it was decided to put the catheter back in. What a relief!

The next day the nurse came and took it out again. Again no luck and more agony. This went on twice more. I did not know what to do as I was told that they were being hopeful. Anyway, I went home with a catheter and was fine about it. I went back after a week to have it removed and it was the worst day of my life. I could pass water but the stinging was getting worse every hour. I was begging for them to do something. By the time the best course of treatment was decided (they were trying to speak to the consultant) I was sent home at

11pm with stronger antibiotics. I felt let down and ready to die. I knew I was in for a painful sleepless night. But was told I needed to let the antibiotics work.

Conclusion: I would take the following before the operation; Uva Ursi is a tincture which helps with UTI's and also arnica is very good for healing the wounds. But nobody told me about the risk of UTI till I got it. Now it is five weeks since and I am on the road to recovery and hope that I can help someone prepare themselves better!

Hope, Mary Dunning

I had my TAH operation on the 20th February 2013 and BSO plus omental biopsy and peritoneal washing. I am awaiting the results from these. I have had problems with my periods most of my life, I suffered from very severe acne as well. I have been experiencing more severe problems over the last five years but was told this was anxiety.

Not sure how I can look six months pregnant with anxiety but generally I found others to be dismissive. However, I had mood changes, bleeding all the time and this was extremely heavy. After being told nothing was wrong I thought I was losing it until I was referred to an excellent consultant.

My message would be to others experiencing problems is to have hope and keep going, be persistent. I was assessed, had bloods taken and a biopsy and most of all she listened to my story which, after five years of knowing there was something wrong was great!

Following this I was told I needed a TAH as a preventative measure as results from tests indicated it was potentially developing into cancer (I had displaced cells) but I'm not sure exactly what this means.

I must say the consultant and medical team I have come into contact with for this surgery have been fantastic! The care and consideration has given me back hope.

When I knew I needed surgery I tried to ignore it and worked very hard so I would not have to think about it. This was due to fear I think! As the date got nearer I realised I had to face my fears and read some research that revealed the importance of preparing both physically and mentally for surgery. It informed me that those individuals who prepared had less blood loss, required less pain relief and recovery was easier. Following this I then prepared by doing more exercise and listening to a CD to prepare for surgery which helped me relax and prepare me mentally for the surgery. I listened to this for 21 days before surgery and am now listening to the post surgery CD to aid my recovery. I also had two hypnosis sessions prior to the surgery to reduce my stress levels (which worked a treat).

On the day of the surgery my husband was amazed at how I kept calm and just got on with it. The consultant told me I had minimal blood loss, I did not need too much pain relief and my recovery has been positive so far. I really believe that the preparation I did was key here, also the medical team made a difficult situation a positive experience.

I am up getting on with life, doing gentle exercises getting fresh air and trying to eat well. I am still off work and not driving yet but hope to be very soon. The support of friends and family is wonderful. If I am truthful I am worried about the results of the tests but want to think positively and realise that personal health and happiness is so, so important.

My recent experiences have made me value the important things in my life and given me faith in the health care professionals. Reading the stories and information on the website has been very useful to me in understanding my own perspective and others. Thank you!

My Journey Of Recovery, Debbie (aged 49 years)

My experience of a full abdominal hysterectomy was not great. Instead of recovering on the gynaecology ward, I was put on the short stay surgical ward where staff were very junior and the experience was very impersonal. I had previously undergone a gynae operation two years ago where things had not gone so well and where I ended up in intensive care. So I was worried about my care already.

I went down for surgery at 1.30pm and remember being in recovery where stabilizing my pain seemed to take some time. I went back to the short stay surgical ward at 6.40pm. There were five other people on the ward and no one else with gynae problems. My husband visited at 7pm for an hour, I was a bit spaced out but remember being pleased to see him. At about 9pm I felt in a lot of pain, was given paracetamol and ibuprofen which had little effect. I tried to rest. The beds emptied leaving me and one other lady in the bay. I was in lots of pain and remember being in tears for some time, eventually an anaesthetist was sent for and I was given some morphine injections, what a relief, managed to sleep.

I woke up to lots of noise. People were being admitted to the other beds for day surgery that day. I asked the time to be told 7.30am. I was a little bit annoyed that I was not feeling too well and was in a bay trying to recover with new people coming in with their relatives waiting for their slot in surgery.

The staff were focused on getting people prepped for day surgery; I might as well have not been there. About 8.30am a lady came round with tea trolley and I got my first hot drink since arriving on Sunday night, it was lovely.

About half an hour later breakfast arrived, I was given orange juice and a Weetabix, ate a little but the pain was back again. Another hour went by and a student nurse took my blood pressure and I asked if anyone was coming to see me, she said a doctor would be up sometime during the day.

I asked for some pain relief she said she would ask. The anaesthetist from the previous night arrived and prescribed me some morphine – thank goodness! The ward continued to be busy with patients being taken up and down to surgery and nursing staff helping these patients. Not a lot happened to me.

In the late afternoon a lady from the surgical team who had operated on me came to see me, said everything went well and that I could go home if I wanted. Horror, here I was on drips, catheters, feeling quite poorly to be told I was okay to go home! I explained that when I came for my pre-op I was told I would be in two to three days at least. I explained that I had no-one to look after me until earliest

Wednesday evening. This was Tuesday about 3pm and she said I could stay till Wednesday!

I was in shock in what I had been told. I know they try to get people home early but this was unbelievable, this was less than 24 hours after the surgery. It felt very impersonal like being in a cattle market. Wow, after the assistant left a nurse came to see me who was really good, and she was able to assure me that I would not be going home until all the drips, catheters and pain relief was managed, plus I needed to see a physiotherapist and get some prescriptions ready for me to take home. The day continued with surgical patients coming and going.

My husband visited again at 7pm, I was so pleased to see him. All the beds were now full of patients, most waiting to be picked up to be taken home from day surgery. The morphine pump helped me a lot throughout the day.

The night staff came on and advised that they were to give me additional saline throughout the night in preparation for me going home tomorrow. I had managed to get in and out of bed, my catheter was removed about tea time but I still had a couple of drips where I needed to wheel the apparatus with the cables and drips around when visiting the toilet. I'm feeling very tired now – just hope I can sleep.

By about 9pm there was only me and one other lady on the ward. Within the next two hours three other people came into the beds and there was lots of activity, one lady was very distressed in particular. Because I was on the saline drip I continually wanted to go to the toilet; this was going to be a busy night! I was feeling in quite a bit of pain due to having to visit the toilet so often and the lady next to me seemed to be very anxious, I managed to calm her down and give her some water as no one was helping her, poor lady!!

So pleased when it started to get light as it had been a long night; more people came onto the ward for surgery again. Here we go again, cannot wait to go home later today.

What I witnessed while in the ward has been shocking! Considering I have worked for the NHS for 27 years I was shocked at the lack of compassion and quality of care! The day goes by, I have my morphine drip taken off me I was told I could take a shower, with no help of course, just get on with it. My stomach is really swollen so cannot see my scar but manage to take my dressings off and clean what I think is my scar. It feels good.

Only a few more hours and I can go home. The patients continue to come into the beds today; these are mostly medical assessment patients where GPs have made referrals with lots of confusion about why, what is expected etc. The staff are not very good at communicating what is going on. One lady has been referred by a GP because she has had diarrhoea and sickness for four days. I was not happy that she was sent to the ward, I did not want to catch anything!

Eventually, all my paperwork is complete so I phone up my husband to come and get me. At 5pm on Wednesday I leave the ward. Hopefully I never have to go in hospital again – what a nightmare! I have observed lots of other things but they are all negative. My questions are why was I not on the gynae ward? Where were the qualified staff? Where was my surgeon? Who is accountable for my care? Is this too much to ask?

Since I have been home things are a lot better, my husband has been great.

Total Hysterectomy, A Fabulous Drama In 3 Weeks! – Dierdra Tara Michelle

On February 27th I partook in the drama of 'A Total Hysterectomy', playing the part of the patient who supplied the uterus, cervix and a couple of sizable tumours that were amorously attached to the aforementioned body parts. I was fortunate to be in a location where a robot was available to assist the able bodied oncologist Dr W, whom I hired to play the part of the doctor. The robot was played by none other than da Vinci, a great mind whom I have always admired from afar, and who rounded out this stellar cast. The alchemy of this cast carried the entire production to a very successful end.

Today, almost three weeks out from this performance, I am a veritable da Vinci poster child! I sport two lovely, giant 'snake bite' marks, puncture wounds paired approximately six inches apart on either side of my waist, a lasting badge for my part in this production.

I am happy beyond happiness for the relief of pain that my body has experienced since accepting its role in 'A Total Hysterectomy'. (Plus I got a bonus piercing in my belly button to boot! Lucky me!)

The hardest part of the entire experience is not being able to jump for joy till the 10 week moratorium on 'freedom of body use' is lifted. Ten weeks of restraint is not too bad for a lifetime of relief and knowing that cancer is not part of my present reality! I will have plenty of days to come to return to a maniac mountain biking, body-working yoga woman, and 'oh yes' my return to SEX.

Before our theatrical production I took the time to honour the sacrifice that my body would make in accepting the award-winning role of hysterectomy recipient. I created a fire-ceremony the night before the 'opening production' in which I expressed my gratitude for all that my uterus and cervix gave me though out my 47 years of life. (In existence at this time, there are three 'Dierdra-spawn' roaming this earth to prove the commitment of the sacrificed body parts to their own beautiful nature!)

Changes are always a bit nerve wracking. My success counted on a part of me to choose to die that I might continue on for whatever years of life are yet to be given to me. As a widow and just as a part of humanity in general, I have learned that whenever there is death, life pumps in a large dose of regenerative energy for those brave enough to stick it through to the other side. I could never say 'Thank You' enough to the Great Cervix and Uterus! (Think Great Pumpkin here!) Every mammal we can think of has passed through you!

In closing I would also like to thank all those around me who made this possible: my beautiful spawn, my fire-keeper and love – Bill, and the countless others who embodied love for me. As I enter back into my vocation of choice, I am sure the lessons learned during the production of 'A Total Hysterectomy' will leak their way into my paintings. Time will tell…for time cannot keep a secret very well! In Gratitude, Love and Happiness. (to be continued …)

Feeling Positive, Helen Clarke

They say we all have a cross to bear, and mine has always been gynae issues. Dodgy smears as a teenager, the agony of endometriosis and finishing off with a fibroid, despite having a Mirena coil fitted to control the endometriosis (Mirena is often the first line of defence to prevent a fibroid increasing in size).

I am 44, have never had kids and had a grapefruit sized fibroid. I opted to have a hysterectomy because my body had been through enough quick fix procedures. It was simply time to take control back of my own body. Reading other stories has made me consider how negative our experiences can be but I wanted to express the positives to anyone about to go through this.

1) Get your head straight. If you can confront the issues of losing your womb before the op you will find it easier to cope afterwards. I always wanted kids, but that is not what life had in store so I took time to prepare my mind. I concentrated on the positives of not having my own children, but being a great auntie to my friends' kids.

2) Talk to friends and family. I was literally astonished by the number of women who said having a hysterectomy was the best thing they had ever done. Not having periods has been liberating for them and more importantly they have been pain free, often after years of suffering.

3) Take it easy. I am three days post-op so I am still in bed, although how long a control freak can put up with hubby doing the cleaning remains to be seen! However, I want this operation to be a long term success and fully intend to rest my body in order to achieve that goal. I have taken up knitting but you might like to learn a language while you have this rare excuse to put your feet up. Learning a new skill will enrich this time, even if I am still constipated, bloated and sore.

The pulsing pain that ran over my abdomen when the epidural wore off is now a distant memory (got to love that Tramadol). In no time at all I will forget I vomited when I tried to pee for the first time post-op. I'm sure the first time my bowels (finally!) move will be a great relief. In the meantime I am looking forward to saying 'my hysterectomy was the best thing I ever did!'

My Story, Best Thing Ever... So Far, Janette Morrison

I started my periods age 10 and had no problems with them. I went on the pill at 16 and was on that for twelve years nonstop until I wanted a baby. I tried for two years and had lots of infertility investigations. Eventually, I did conceive and had a son 21 years ago by c-section. I was very ill after spending five days on life support following a problem with the anaesthetic. I have had several abnormal smear tests and had laser treatment and cone biopsy.

I had continued to have problems with periods on and off since then having tried the medications which worked but made me feel drunk and not myself at all. I tried a coil but didn't get on with that either. This year I have had two separate month-long really heavy and painful periods which resulted in me becoming severely anaemic requiring iron transfusions and I got to the point where I had had enough. I had to have various other blood tests, investigations and procedures to eliminate other causes of anaemia.

I then had a gynae consult and a uterine biopsy. He agreed that a laparoscopic hysterectomy was the way forward. I was very wary, not because of op and relief it would give me, but the anaesthetic due to past problems. I met with the consultant anaesthetist who reassured me so I was given a date of 21st December 2012.

Although not ideal being on top of Christmas I accepted the date as hubby is off for 10 days from work anyway so no extra help would be needed.

However the biopsy was abnormal, I was told on the 13th November and had the op on 14th so was in shock, understandably so.

It all went very well, I tried to be positive and think of the benefits thinking 2013 was going to be MY year.

I came home on 16th November and have been pleasantly surprised by how *well* I feel. I miss not being able to sleep on my tummy (too sore), I miss walking my doggie and I miss having a bath. I have been given different timescales for these things to re-commence. On the plus side I lost 5lbs post-op and the pain and bleeding is much better than what I had been suffering. I am hoping to continue to improve this way and wishing everyone else well with their operation and recovery.

Finally The Pain Has Gone, Karen Peacock

I was diagnosed at 29 with severe endometriosis. I was told if I had been 10 years older and had a family they would have done a hysterectomy then! Due to my age and having no family it was difficult to treat and over the years I had various non invasive treatments including seven laparoscopies, Synarel, the pill, contraceptive injections, coil etc. I would get a few months relief then it would all return.

Over the past year my quality of life has been affected, almost constant pain affecting my day to day schedule including work, exercise etc.

In October I went for my three monthly visit to the consultant and was given an ultimatum; continue with non invasive treatments for the next 8-10 years or have a hysterectomy! Not the easiest decision I have had to make! I had a week to make my decision and armed with a list of questions I went to see consultant again.

My decision was to have a hysterectomy. I had lived with this horrible condition for 12 years and had enough! So aged 41 without a family (there are other options) I had TAH/BSO on 9th January. Despite a few initial problems post-op and being re-admitted to hospital, I am now just over five weeks post-op and whilst not fully recovered, I feel better now than I have done in years and know I have made the right decision. I am now looking forward to a healthy and pain free 2013.

Early Days, Kate Hulm

My fibroids were first diagnosed in July 2006 and as the rather stark information from my GP was either have a hysterectomy or do nothing, I decided to do nothing. I felt I would rather cope with heavy periods than have a major operation – who wouldn't?

A year later after becoming progressively more uncomfortable and not realising that the majority of my issues would be fibroid related, a helpful, awareness raising email was the final straw. I convinced myself I had ovarian cancer as all the symptoms listed were my symptoms and I knew that my ovaries had not been visible in the original scan. Luckily I was able to have another scan very quickly (but privately) which showed that I had a veritable garden of fibroids, with a magnificent centre piece and healthy ovaries.

A referral to a consultant swiftly followed but again using private medical insurance. My consultant was lovely and I learned about the variety of options that could help treat my condition. However, her recommendation was to have a hysterectomy as my largest fibroid was a significant size (8cm) and she felt that other options might result in further complications. I had two Zoladex injections, four weeks apart, to induce a temporary menopause in order to shrink the large fibroid and make the surgery less invasive (a horizontal rather than vertical incision).

Despite 'going privately' the date of my surgery was delayed a week, which was probably one of the most stressful weeks of my life. We duly presented ourselves at the appointed time (7am!!) on Wednesday 28th November. There is a slightly surreal feeling about going to have an operation, particularly a fairly major one, when you actually don't feel so bad. The Zoladex had improved many of my symptoms, most significantly the pain in my pelvis and my lack of bladder control, although had done nothing to control the almost constant bleeding I was experiencing.

I had to wait until 10am (which I do recognise is not very long but felt like eternity as I was so agitated) to go down to theatre. My other half caught forty winks in the rather uncomfortable hospital chair due to our early start, while I manically Sudoku'd my way through the three hour wait! Oh for the days of pre-meds!

The theatre staff, consultant included, were very nice but all I could think was 'let's get this over and done with'! I had been told or read about what would happen during the operation but I am a bit of an ostrich when it comes to wanting to know about people rummaging around inside me while I am asleep, not to mention what they do to your external anatomy to make the operation more hygienic from their point of view! The next thing I knew I was coming too in recovery in agony. Luckily a good friend who had had a c-section with her second child had told me how much this would hurt (no one else had) and also how quickly it would recede with the PCA, which it did.

The operation had taken about two hours and I was in recovery for about two more. Needless to say the rest of Wednesday passed in a blur for me, I tried to talk to my very concerned looking husband but it was all a bit of an effort and not very scintillating! Same husband brought our children in later on Wednesday evening and my daughter promptly burst into tears. All the tubes attached to various bits of my anatomy were a bit scary to see but probably no scarier than her imagination and at 10 years old perhaps starting to see real life is no bad thing. My 13 year old son was outwardly more stoic but did ask my husband some difficult questions when they got home like 'Can anything go wrong now?'

I did not sleep well the first night in hospital (or any other night for that matter) despite or perhaps because of the morphine. The nursing staff were very gentle and kind and my first cup of tea (in a sippy cup like a toddler just in case you doze off in the middle of drinking) was incredibly wonderful. I had been given some Japanese peppermint oil by a friend who had had a hysterectomy in the summer. I began drinking it that night, two drops in a small amount of warm water, to combat the dreaded wind that everyone had said was likely to be the worst thing about being post-op. I actually never thought this; my bruised and battered internal organs and lower tummy were, and remain, more painful.

Early Thursday morning my catheter was removed and by lunchtime I was in agony with urine retention, a fairly common complication, and had to be re-catheterised for a further 24 hours, an undignified process but an indescribable relief. On Friday getting out of bed seemed like a huge step forward and after I had done it with assistance a couple of times I could do it by myself very carefully. Saturday was my day to weep, again I think a very normal reaction to the trauma of operation both physical and emotions. The staff were all very kind and allowed me to cry myself dry and happier. Sunday was D-day and although very sore and achy I was pleased to be going home. I made the mistake of kneeling down in the bathroom and had to call for assistance to get me back up on my feet – it is quite amazing what tummy muscles actually do.

I am writing this having been home for nearly a week – an attentive partner or friend is essential to recovery, I can do very little – and recognise how much improved I am from this time last week. Still tired, sore and stiff but able to move more easily and think coherently again. Visits from friends are a lifeline to the real world and planning things in the future to look forward to (we have booked tickets to see Bruce Springsteen next June, a lifelong ambition of mine, as a result of all the radio listening in hospital).

Everyone I know who has had a hysterectomy says it was the best thing they did and while there is little to recommend the process, we are so lucky in our country to have options and good hospitals and surgeons. I am now eagerly anticipating the 'new woman' I have been told I will become in due course and plan to make this as positive a life changing event as I possibly can.

Total Hysterectomy, Kerry Farrell

I had a total abdominal hysterectomy on 21st November 2012, I should have had a vaginal but there were complications as my bladder was attached to my bowel and my pelvic wall and had to be cut away in a four hour op.

I woke up in agony – the morphine drip made me very sick so didn't have it and I ended up on Paracetamol which didn't touch the pain.

I had to have catheter fitted for 10 days which was uncomfortable. I got a really bad bladder infection and it hurt really badly when I peed, my bowels were not particularly good either.

I had my ovaries removed and am now on HRT. I'm quite emotional and down as I'm still in a lot of pain. I'm normally a very active person and find it hard and draining getting through the day. I've got a wonderful supportive partner who has been fab and nursing me back to good health.

One Week After Total Abdominal Hysterectomy, Donna Emery

Hi. I had a total abdominal hysterectomy (TAH) last Tuesday afternoon. The op was apparently tricky because of the severity of my endometriosis and the cyst (8.4cm) that was on my right ovary had attached itself to the wall of my body making it tricky to part with.

The consultant had to remove my uterus, tubes, ovaries and cervix, so when I came back onto the ward I was in a lot of pain. But luckily the morphine pump was on hand. I was kept on oxygen all night and at 2am they called the doctor to query the amount of blood that I had lost. I was borderline having a transfusion but luckily all was okay.

The next day they removed my morphine pump in the morning and catheter in the afternoon. Getting up for the first time was scary although it wasn't as bad as I thought it was going to be. I managed to get up and about a few times to go to the bathroom and felt really proud of myself!!

The drain came out in the evening. Ouchy!

I kept myself quite active the next day doing laps around the nurses' station, was hoping it would help with sleeping too!!

On the Friday I had to have a scan where I had dye put through me to check that my kidneys were not damaged, once again all was fine.

Six days after the op I have had my stitches out. I feel okay. I am walking around quite well and the stairs are getting easier. The first bowel movement made me hit the roof, but apart from that each day gets a lot easier and I'm only on paracetamol now for the pain!!

My advice to anyone about to go through it is take each day as it comes, never expect too much and be proud of your achievements.

Shell Shocked After Giving Birth, Kerry Robinson

I was admitted to hospital to be induced with my second baby thinking that I'd be discharged again about six hours after the birth, I wrong was I.

After giving birth to my little girl naturally the midwife went to sew up where they'd had to cut me and noticed I was bleeding quite heavily. The next thing I knew the room was full of people and I was being rushed to surgery.

When I woke up in intensive care the next day my husband told me that they had had to perform a hysterectomy to save my life as there was no other way of stopping the bleeding.

I didn't really know how to feel about it and three weeks on I'm still not sure. My husband and I had already decided that we wouldn't be having anymore children after this pregnancy anyway but to have the final decision taken away from me at the age of 32 is heart breaking.

Physically I'm recovering okay. I have been told that they managed to save my ovaries. But when I went for a scan yesterday to check that everything is going back to where it should be they could only find my right ovary. So I'm now waiting to hear back from my consultant. Other than that my wound has healed nicely although it is still numb but tender if that makes sense. I still feel quite sore in my lower abdomen and still have some bleeding.

Emotionally I feel like I'm on a roller coaster as one day I think I'm doing okay and the next I'm in tears.

Unfortunately I was discharged from hospital with very little information about the hysterectomy as I was primarily cared for on maternity wards so the site has been invaluable when I've had questions. For example nine days after the op I passed two massive blood clots which scared me beyond belief. I went to A&E to be checked out and it turns out it's normal to pass some clots, if only I'd known that!

It's still early days for me getting my head round having the hysterectomy but I can honestly say that physically I don't feel that bad.

Looking Forward To The Rest Of My Life! Lisa

Since Monday 18th March I have ventured forth in the adventure that is the rest of my life! My menstrual problems began after a post-partum haemorrhage following the birth of our second child; a natural delivery of a 10lb 6oz bouncing baby boy! My cycle went from accurate to irregular. I went on to have our third child, another boy but only 9lbs 10oz this time! Menstruation resumed irregularly and that became my life. Carrying a second set of clothes to work became the norm, sitting and then standing fearing flooding and then the duration of this became longer until latterly I used to get four days off between cycles! I became seriously anaemic HB dropped to 5.2 so needed a transfusion and then they started investigations.

Firstly I had a polyp removed and then the Mirena coil fitted. The 'grappling hook' fell out after three months and then a second fell out after four weeks. Then I had an ablation which didn't stop the flow but reduced it considerably.

All was good for six months and then it started again with bouts of anaemia and virtually constant bleeding. I was referred back and thankfully saw my fabulous gynaecologist again. He worked his magic removing my womb, ovaries and cervix. My womb was the size of a 16 week pregnancy and full of fibroids! Better out than in don't you think?

I am in my third week since the op and from the moment I came round from the anaesthetic I haven't looked back. I am being a very good girl, doing as I'm told and taking things steady! I feel like a new woman and I feel blessed. I am thankful for my surgeon's expertise and experience and for enabling me to live the rest of my life free from pain and anaemia. The nurses were fabulous as nothing was too much trouble and after some of the experiences I had read about here I was quite nervous about that.

I realise that this may not be everyone's situation and I am very fortunate in that we have three great teenagers and so I haven't the psychological trauma aspect of the hysterectomy taking away my hopes of having a family. But if you are facing this don't be scared or fearful, I was and thought I wouldn't wake up from the anaesthetic.

It will change your life but if your situation is like mine it will change it for the better. Looking forward to convalescing, the lifting of the six week embargo and a phased return to work after 12 weeks and I'm still excited about going to the toilet for just a wee without any mess etc. pathetic I know but it's been years!

Heavy Periods, My Post-Op Story, Steph Powell

I am now 10 days post-op. Arrived at the hospital 25th March at 7am on a very snowy Monday morning, had spent all weekend worrying that my op would be cancelled again, due to the bad weather, but luckily the phone didn't ring.

After checking in and sitting in the waiting room with my mom for company - my partner had to work - for a couple of hours we finally got called in to see the consultant who explained the operation and answered questions. After that we saw the anaesthetist I can still remember her saying that when you come round you'll be in no pain, but you will know you have had surgery. I wondered what she meant but didn't question it. Finally we saw the ward sister who did all the final checks, blood, urine ECG etc. whilst this was being completed a nurse popped her head around the door to say they were ready for me in theatre.

Up until now I was surprised at how calm I had been feeling, but now I couldn't even get the ties on my gown done up, had to ask my mom for help, surgical stockings were another problem, after about fifteen minutes I was finally ready, with a hug from mom and accompanied by a nurse I made the long walk to theatre.

Once there the anaesthetist was very calming and before I knew it I was under. On coming round all I could feel was an immense pain in my abdomen, I was in so much pain I somehow kicked my catheter out, my heart rate became erratic and I was shivering uncontrollably. Apparently I was having a reaction to the anaesthetic. I was put back to sleep whilst they sorted out my catheter and pain control.

When I woke again I was back on the ward feeling much more comfortable, still in a little pain but the morphine pump sorted that out and boy did I enjoy pushing that button! The next few hours passed in a blur with half hour observations and the nurses constantly asking me about my level of pain, I couldn't praise the nurses enough, nothing was ever too much for them.

My mom and partner arrived for evening visiting and by then I was fully awake and having fun playing with the bed controls! After visiting I was surprised at how well and awake I felt, spent the time talking to the two other women who were in the small four bed bay with me.

Around midnight I started itching very badly down below, knowing I was allergic to latex I called the nurse who quickly examined me and agreed that the catheter needed to come out. I was a little nervous about this but actually I didn't feel a thing and as soon as it was out I instantly felt the need to pee so a commode was fetched as I was still attached to the morphine pump so couldn't move far from the bed.

Took a little while for things to start flowing but once they did it was such a relief as I had heard so many stories about women having problems in this department.

The rest of the night and next day flew by, I was out of bed the minute the morphine was finished and at 10am Tuesday morning was having a strip wash by my bedside and into clean underwear and pj's all completed unaided and painlessly. The consultant came to see me before lunch and was amazed at my activity and best of all agreed I could go home as soon as meds etc. were sorted. Had lessons on how to do my anti blood clot injections before I left, have to inject once a day for 10 days.

Arrived home around 6pm that Tuesday evening. A day after after surgery and I haven't looked back since. I feel very very lucky, because unlike a lot of ladies my pain has been minimal and I am already down to only taking pain killers twice a day. Because I am feeling so good, the fact that I must allow my body to heal and rest is the only cure, I am becoming frustrated at my lack of being able to do anything. During the last few days I have limited myself to making drinks for myself and my partner and loading and emptying the washing machine together with a little light dusting.

My scar is looking very good and I have to admit I am quite proud of it. I had dissolving stitches with steri-strips on top. The strips were taken off on Tuesday by the nurse at my local surgery and I am now allowed to bath and shower. Today is my last injection which is nice because we are running out of space to do them, some for some reason they tend to leave a big nasty bruise whereas others just leave a pin prick mark!

It's been a relatively short journey for me, from being diagnosed with fibroids in November 2012 to having my op March 2013, but happily I now start my new period free life and what a relief.

To all those ladies waiting for surgery I am sending big gentle hugs, as you can see from my story it's not all scary hospitals, mega pain stories, with cold uncaring nurses looking after you, I was very lucky in that my initial pain was sorted quickly and the nurses that looked after me obviously love their job and care about their patients. Since coming out of hospital I have done very well, maybe my positive attitude has a lot to do with that, but then again maybe it's all down to the amazing surgeon I had, whatever the answer I know a lot of ladies won't be as fortunate as me and that saddens me. But as long as you stay positive there is light at the end of the hysterectomy tunnel, stay positive.

Not Out Of The Woods But There Is Improvement, Carmen

First of all let me explain how this came about. I had been suffering with numbness in my toes for quite some time and was getting quite concerned that I might have something neurologically wrong which may be causing these symptoms. After visiting a chiropodist and a physiotherapist I went back to my doctor and requested referral to a hospital. I got my referral and this resulted in an MRI scan.

The MRI scan was on the lower lumber region as well as neck. The lower lumber region scan showed up a large mass in my pelvic area which sent my original issue to the back burner as the mass took priority and had to be investigated further.

I then went to a different hospital and had another MRI scan, along with ultrasound and a physical internal examination. The consultant then told me I had what she believed to be a dermoid cyst; she explained that when she gave me the internal examination she felt bone!

I was horrified when she told me that a dermoid is a sort of growth of what could be components of a human being. It could contain the following.

Mature skin complete with hair follicles and sweat glands, sometimes clumps of long hair, and often pockets of sebum, blood, fat, bone, nails, teeth, eyes, cartilage, and thyroid tissue.

I was in much distress having had this news, I actually said to the nurse when dressing I have a monster inside me! I had no idea this thing lurked within me over God knows how many years. I had suffered bouts of tenderness in the left ovary region and also when having sex I could feel pain if my partner went in a too deep. I put it down to perhaps a bit of IBS?

My consultant contacted me and confirmed it was a dermoid and then gave me an option to go for the removal with a full abdominal hysterectomy along with removal of the ovaries to avoid further issues.

I must admit I didn't give it a great deal of thought, being 55 I had gone past wanting any children, these organs weren't any use to me really, they may as well all come out. So I agreed to the FAB with a bikini cut.

I found after I made the decision the closer the operation was getting the more emotional I was becoming, the fear that things can go wrong and I may not survive this, even though statistically the odds of me not surviving were low I still worried about it. I guess as you get older these things are more to the forefront.

These thoughts really did challenge me – I was pretty low and wept many times. I was so convinced of the possibility of not coming back that I actually pinned down a solicitor the day before my operation and made a will. I wrote letters to my loved ones, which was really difficult; it was like staring at your past and having to revisit painful places saying sorry to those you may have hurt. I got my documents in order, contacted pension companies to verify my next of kin and basically left instructions. It all sounds very morbid now but me being Miss Organized it was my natural path.

The day of the operation I took myself to the hospital and faced it head on, to my amazement I was no sooner checking in to being on a surgery trolley, it was so fast as I was the first operation of the afternoon. I expected to be taken to the ward first and be prepared from there. That's not how it works anymore.

The nurse's that looked after me were brilliant – we had a few jokes and they put me at ease. I was given an injection in my spine and also the full on anaesthetic that takes you out totally.

I was in surgery two hours. I recall coming round and not being able to feel my legs which did alarm me because the guy that was wheeled in after me was moving his feet. I said to the angel that was watching over me (the post-op nurse) 'I can't feel my legs?' He reassured me and said 'It's fine Carmen they will come back, this is normal.' I am glad to say they did eventually. I was wheeled back on ward by 7pm. I had no ill effects from the anaesthetic, in fact by 8pm I was hungry, but I wasn't allowed to eat until the following day.

I also found I was wide awake for most of the night, I had a morphine button which I tried not to use too often, I tried to restrict the use to six hour gaps, afterwards I realized it was drip feeding into me all the time, the button was just for when the pain was worse.

I took my laptop into hospital so that I could watch DVDs and listen to my music otherwise the boredom would have driven me nuts, and no way was I paying £10.00 a day for the use of a TV.

It was very hard to sleep in hospital because our ward served as an A&E ward, the lights were on all of the time, and it could get noisy so I would advise anyone going in to take an eye mask and earplugs. Having said that I think I had a wide awake reaction to the morphine. I couldn't believe it – I am a sleepy person generally; I usually doze off by 9pm on my sofa at home.

I was advised that I had slight bleeding, a trickle on the inner wall of the vagina so they inserted some packing to help this wound to clot.

On day one post-op I was given a bed bath and also the packing that was inserted into my vagina needed to be removed. Nothing prepared me for this. I was expecting maybe at best a six inch swab; it turned out to feel like 20 inches. I said to the nurse 'Are you going to pull out some coloured scarves and a rabbit?' It felt very odd to say the least.

On day two I rose out of bed and had my first wee which was followed by three number two's!

I think the frequency of the number 2's was as a result of the hospital food, which was awful – I wouldn't have given the first meal I was served to a dog. After that I stuck to salads.

Believe me having a poo felt like a milestone the whole ward got to know about. At the time you are so worried about straining, because you can't push for fear of damaging yourself.

Day three I managed to have a shower which was heaven, being able to wash my hair and feel sort of self-sufficient again. The walk to and from the bathroom was a long shuffle but the reward at the end of it was worth it.

On the morning of day four I was discharged. It felt wonderful putting some clothes on and shuffling to the fresh air. I will say standing up felt very odd. I felt and still feel a weightiness in my tummy, I guess what has been left behind is still swollen.

It was lovely to get home and to climb into my big soft comfy bed; the tranquillity of the silence in my little flat was so comforting.

My disappointment seven days on was that I have gone on the scales and my weight is exactly the same. I would have thought the removal of a dermoid the size of a tennis ball, two ovaries and a womb would at least weigh 4lbs!

My shame is that I can't bring myself to look at the wound, it feels fine and I was told it was healing perfectly, in fact the duty ward doctor asked whose work it was, like it was a painting. I just can't bring myself to look at it.

Day eight I start to see some light coloured pinky blood and a brown discharge which alarmed me so I searched for information on the internet and found this lovely support group. I also contacted my doctor and made an appointment for this coming Wednesday for a check-up.

Yesterday which was day 11 post-surgery I changed the bedding on my bed, it exhausted me. I was told off for doing this by many of my friends on Facebook. I also took a short walk which felt very liberating; it was such a lovely day it was wasted being indoors.

There is no doubt post-op is a long haul; thank God for the internet which is proving to be my healing buddy.

I was finding as the days progressed I was feeling more and more unwell. I sort of expected hot flushes as the operation had sent me into a menopausal downward spiral, however I was finding I was experiencing chills and fever like symptoms. I found that no matter how many quilts and blankets I would cover myself up with I was extremely cold, shivering in fact. I wasn't prepared for this and eventually felt I needed to go and see my GP. It took me a number of days to get an appointment but eventually I got to see her.

When I arrived in her office I was in such a state both physically and mentally I found as soon as I tried to explain how I felt floods of tears came out. I guess it was the relief of telling someone how awful and desperate I felt, remember I was going through this alone and the preceding days of isolation and feeling so ill sort of caught up with me. The first thing she did was take my temperature, and then she took it again. She then said she was going to write a letter and that I needed to take the letter with me to the assessment ward at the hospital. I phoned for a taxi and went there straight away.

I was only wearing a thin coat and finding it very cold; they put me on a bed-type trolley and placed me in an area where curtains separated each patient. They kept taking my temperature and blood pressure along with blood samples for what seemed like hours, meanwhile I shivered. I kept asking for a blanket but they wouldn't give me one. I couldn't understand why they wouldn't give me a simple blanket. A nurse explained that they had to bring my temperature down so a blanket was not an option.

Eventually a doctor came and looked at the readings and listened to my symptoms and then told me what was wrong with me. He said I had gone what is known as 'septic'. He immediately admitted me to be assigned the next available bed in the assessment ward. I was hooked up to a machine that was feeding me some sort of fluid; I waited for at least another two hours and eventually got on the ward and put to bed. I was so shocked that I had ended up back in hospital, at the time I didn't realise how serious this was, this was life threatening, my body temperature was through the roof. I never thought of taking my temperature at home at anytime. Something so simple should have alerted me to get to a hospital straight away.

I was continually fed antibiotics by drip for the next few days.

On day three of my second admittance I felt well enough to go and have a shower. I limped up to the shower room had my shower and started to walk back to my bed. I sat on the bed and was talking to the lady in the next bed, and then all of a sudden I felt a burst of fluid, and all of this Barbie pink coloured stuff appears on my brand new white linen nightdress and on the floor. It was major panic around me as I stood dripping this weird coloured fluid, I was so frightened and the poor nurse was in shock trying to think of what to do. Another more experienced nurse came and sat me down, she then went and got a bag and sort of attached it to the leaking area – I think they use these bags to drain fluids. She then taped a large dressing over the top. Basically I had developed what is known as a haematoma, a collection of fluid beneath my wound and the fluid burst through my wound.

The assessment ward contacted the gynaecology ward and made them aware of the incident, which then lead to me being transferred to the ward where I had had my hysterectomy. I was so relieved to be placed in their care. I knew many of the nurses and they made me feel so welcome and cared for.

I had found the assessment ward so cold and clinical – you had every combination of illness in there.

One lady had Alzheimer's continually thinking she was being burgled and shouting in the night. I also recall a lady that was allowed to sleep in her chair for 2 nights, her legs and face were so badly burned the chair held the most comfort for her.

But what upset me most of all, and it makes me cry to recall it, was an old lady opposite me who was the image of my mother. Her hair was pure white and so thick, she was so small I could have put my index figure and thumb around her wrist and still have room – she was so terribly thin and fragile and looked in distress many times. She kept trying to take her clothes off because she was hot and she also was showing signs of stress by threaded a comfort blanket through her hands continually whilst her eyes were shut. It was so sad to witness her like this; she must have been a seamstress at one time, feeding cloth. It really did upset me to see her so helpless and me being unable to walk to her bed to give her comfort in such a cold environment. It was like she was my mum and I couldn't help her, caged in a bed frame. Both Deb, the lady in the bed next to me, and I kept a close eye on her and alerted the nurses to show her some care and attention when she lost her blanket. Thankfully she had a very attentive relative who would call on her many times through the day.

I had formed a great friendship with Deb on the assessment ward – she gave me so much strength and warmth as we both went through a very trying time, she made light of situations and made me laugh whilst all around me things looked so depressing and helpless.

Yes I was glad to see the back of the assessment ward, but sad to leave Deb behind, she was such a lovely woman. I later realized how unselfish she was. Deb was very ill; she was released from hospital and came to visit me before she went home with her partner Michelle, to then be readmitted a few weeks later. I did go and see her on the ward, she looked awful, so tired, she had bowel cancer and I am sad to say it took her a few weeks later.

I was back on the gynaecology ward, and put on the emergency surgery list to have my wound drained, I was placed on nil by mouth for a whole day waiting to be operated on and then carried forward to the following morning, to then be removed from the waiting list by another doctor who felt it was unnecessary, her words were, 'This wound is draining naturally.' I was kept in for a total of six nights, fed antibiotics on a drip and then released to the care of the district nurses.

I can't express how wonderful it felt to be home, in my own bed and in such a quiet calm environment and to have some decent food. The nurses would come every day for the next two months packing my wound. I still felt very much out of control in that I would never know when they would come. I was a prisoner in my own home; my days consisted of waiting for the nurse, sleeping and web browsing. I also found that I was receiving conflicting status reports on my wounds – it felt like one step forward two steps back many times, I lost count how many different antibiotics I was placed on. I gradually found that my walking was getting better and my strength/stamina was improving so I decided to take control and make a big decision of going back to work on a phased return. I had been off just over five months and my savings were depleting. I had to earn some money – the SSP hand out wouldn't even cover my rent.

When I advised the district nurse of my intentions she immediately released me from their care saying that I was now mobile and needed to be transferred to the walk-in centre for daily dressing changes in the afternoon, which is where I am at now. It's very tedious and I do get the feeling of being dumped by the district nurse team leader because I have no fixed appointments. Sometimes I have to wait more than an hour with what appears to all walks of life having varying ailments and bugs around me, but at least it's a sort of structure to my day and gives me a feeling of having some control of my day-to-day life again. Unfortunately since in their care I have been told the last swab result revealed I had contracted the MRSA bacteria, which has resulted in my being placed on another antibiotic.

I am wondering if this bacteria has been inside me for some time; it would explain why I have taken so long to heal and the many different antibiotics not working so far? What I am struggling to comprehend is that my care has not changed as a result of having this bacteria, I expected to be quarantined thinking this was dangerous to others in the walk-in centre's care. But nothing has changed!

I am hoping the next swab results show that the infection is clear. I have a holiday planned with my mum soon, she is totally unaware that all of this has happened to me and is probably wondering why I have kept away from her for almost a year now. I may have to tell her if my wound is still open and I need to dress it myself.

I am now at 1cm open.

The good thing is the pain in my left side appears to be subsiding and the swelling has lessened. I have found that sometimes I feel like something is clinging onto my bowel, but pain killers ease the pain.

I have been told this could be scar tissue. I have an ultrasound in three weeks which I hope makes the picture clearer.

On a positive note I can now dance more and feel physically stronger. I still require monster sleeps in the afternoon and that's five months on. What I have learned is to never expect a good day will result in another good day following it. I still feel I am not out of the woods but there is improvement be it slow.

My aim is to have a damn good holiday with mum and return back to work full time in mid April.

Just By Chance, Gail

Hi my name is Gail and I am 47. I am currently four weeks post-op from having a hysterectomy with everything removed ovaries, tubes, womb and cervix. It all started around 18-24 months ago. My husband had fallen ill with M.E. my mother and father came to live with us, my father had physical problems and my kids had caring needs.

I took myself to the docs and asked if she could do me a physical check-up as my family were all ill and I needed to maintain that I was well, at this point I was having bowel problems which was put down to irritable bowel syndrome and was given meds. However, on examination of my tummy the doctor told me I had an enlarged womb and referred me to the hospital for a scan. The result was I had two fibroids, one was 5cm and one was around 2.5cms. I was also anaemic as my periods were heavy which I had put down to my age; only to be told by the doctor it wasn't due to my age. I was given iron tablets.

The decision from the hospital was to give me the Mirena coil as the fibroids would disappear when I was in the change. I had the coil fitted and when I went for my check-up the threads were not visible so off I went for another scan, the coil was in place however it had gone up into my cervix.

I persevered with the coil hoping that it would stop my periods or at least slow the heaviness down. However, 12 months in I found I was wearing a pad every day. Not that it was heavy but it was always present. One day I passed a small clot so I took myself off to the doctors again as I thought I might be pregnant again and wanted to check the coil hadn't moved. The GP sent me for another scan and I was told 'there is your cyst'. I immediately said 'what cyst?'

It was on my ovaries and was around 2-3cms, this was not present on my previous scan. The doctor gave me a vaginal scan to have a closer look at the cyst. The next thing the GP requested a blood test to rule out ovarian cancer as the scan was inconclusive; this was unreal so I never really got to grips with what was happening.

I never heard anything from the blood test which was positive, however I was no longer happy with what was happening as I had come about the enlarged womb, the fibroids and the cyst by chance and there was no mention of monitoring the cyst so I requested to be referred back to the hospital.

At the appointment they arranged to do a scrape to clean out the womb and hopefully stop the periods for a while or slow them down. I went in for the procedure, there was a lot of pulling and tugging and that was just to remove the coil! Then they carried on, after about an hour they abandoned the procedure as the fibroids were pressing close to my cervix meaning they couldn't gain entry.

My only other option was to have a hysterectomy that would take everything. The doctor didn't want to leave me with my ovaries to have to come back with another problem at a later date. I agreed.

At this time I couldn't eat properly as I felt full all the time, and I looked six months pregnant. I was put on the waiting list and within three months I had the op.

Everything went okay although the pain afterwards shocked me a little, never having a caesarean, however I persevered.

Up until now I have not decided whether to take HRT as I did have a suspected blood clot scare two weeks post-op; I am not sure whether I would be able to go on it. The good thing is that although my bowels are still not working perfectly I have had no irritable bowel symptoms.

They told me my womb was the size of a 16 week foetus, which was obviously taking considerable space. I can now eat a full meal and enjoy (not) the hot flushes.

The doctor has signed me off work for 12 weeks and I am just starting to go out; it's tiring but I will make progress daily. I do not feel at a loss, I have had five children and five grand kids so I do not want anymore. I just hope my mood continues to be as stable as it is which is much better than it was when I had all my bits.

Light At The End Of The Tunnel, Louise

I am 46 and post hysterectomy.

The website helped me enormously and as did the book advertised on it. I especially liked the new perfume and comfort cushion tips both of which I had already done before I read the book. I would like to share my experience as it is a positive one and it seems there are so many women having to go through so many hoops to secure a satisfactory outcome.

I only went to the Dr about my symptoms two months ago. I had experienced heavy periods for years but put this down to my age. I found I was in discomfort when I stooped to put my shoes on or went to sleep. So that was why I originally went. I now realise that I was suffering with a lot more for years.

I was referred immediately to have an ultrasound as the GP felt what he described was a six month pregnancy uterus. I was definitely not pregnant but I had to have a pregnancy test. The ultrasound was the following week and confirmed large fibroids in the uterus and a 17cm in diameter complex cyst on my ovary which sat so high it gave the impression of pregnancy. It was up to my ribs and had been there for years slowly growing.

So then they tested me for pancreatic and ovarian cancer. This was a big shock just before Christmas and was devastating to my three children (aged 19, 23 and 26). Even when you get the results back, that feeling never quite goes away as you are told that until the cysts and fibroids are removed and biopsies are done cancer cannot be ruled out completely.

So the next thing was a gynae appointment and an MRI to confirm the size. A month had passed since the ultrasound and the MRI showed the cyst had grown 2cms. So my hysterectomy was booked in and a month later I was in and out of hospital. I had a vertical incision and I am not expecting to get over this quickly which I think is realistic. But I will listen to my body and know when I am able to do a bit more. I have not had any bleeding and am not going to miss the sanitary/tampon scene! I am now waiting for my histology results and to go back for my two week check-up.

The consultant told me my growths weighed over 7lbs so no wonder I was struggling. I won't lie; I was in pain for a couple of days after and was reassured this was due to my intestines adjusting to the space etc. The nurses were brilliant and caring and my whole experience has been a positive one.

I was warned that I would be thrust into menopause but so far I feel okay. Just a bit 'away with the fairies' but I am no longer taking medication of any kind and thank my lucky stars. So please do not fear. I have met so many women whilst in hospital and we have all been swapping notes.

I would just like to say that remember menopause is a natural state for all women and not an illness. I have rarely been to the doctor's in my life except while I was pregnant and do not have a history of anything so this experience for me has been life changing. I am so fortunate that my uterus and ovaries served me well indeed and I have three amazing children who are now waiting on me hand and foot.

Two Weeks After, Trish Williams

Hi, I'm Tricia and mine's a flavoured earl grey or vodka and lemonade depending on the time of day!

Four years ago aged 57 I had surgery for breast cancer. Up until the surgery I was having regular monthly periods then BAM! straight into menopause and I wondered what had hit me.

My hysterectomy two weeks ago, removing tubes and ovaries, was as a result of a 'grossly enlarged womb' for which I had a hysteroscopy in August this year. I was still bleeding from this surgery last month when the consultant strongly recommended I have an urgent hysterectomy. I literally had one week from him suggesting it and the surgery.

Fortunately I am retired and my husband is looking after me very well. I went out for a short, slow walk today for the first time. I have been in no pain but my tummy is still sore. I am doing my exercises but only twice a day not three times.

I do wonder about HRT because my cancer was oestrogen sensitive but I do feel I am going to need something to get me back to 'my old self'.

Hysterectomy wasn't on my bucket list but I am glad to have had the surgery so I can get back to yoga and fast walking. How impressed am I that I am no longer bleeding! Yes it was scary but I think listen to your body and be sensible. So glad I came across the website. Thanks.

Happy Silver Wedding Anniversary! Susan

I am 48 years old, have one daughter and have never, ever suffered from any real gynae problems. I had my appendix out in my early teens and it turned out the pain they thought was appendicitis was actually a mid-cycle pain caused by ovulation. However, although I suffered this intermittently through my life it was never a problem and I would only become aware of it if I allowed myself to get over-tired or did too much.

I have always been a very active and mostly fit and healthy person. In this last year I suffered a bad case of food poisoning which took a stone off my weight (which was never too high) and once recovered I felt very well but was thin. My periods have continued as normal and were every four weeks on the dot and have remained the same, slightly lighter in the last year or so. No menopausal symptoms to note only suffering night sweats the night before my period started which has been the same all my life.

In the middle of July I experienced pain in my lower left abdomen and just thought it was the ovulation pain, We had been very busy with a wedding and then I had guests staying so much cooking, cleaning, bed changing etc. and one of the guests was a six month baby whom I spent a lot of time lifting and carrying around. However, this time the pain was a bit different and lasted much longer than the usual day. I also felt tired and was a bit constipated (very unusual for me). After two weeks I thought I should see my GP and the night before my appointment felt a significant lump in my lower abdomen which hadn't been there before. I thought it might be because my bowel had backed up.

I went to see my GP the following afternoon. He did an abdominal examination and should never play poker for a living – his face showed real shock on feeling the lump! He then said he wanted me back first thing the following morning to have bloods taken and was immediately referring me for an ultrasound. He was going to phone the local hospital after my appointment and would let me know when I could be seen when I came back for the bloods to be taken. He was very nice and asked if I was frightened/worried but explained one of the blood tests would be for ovarian cancer. He did all this with compassion and took time to talk to me and asked me to come the next day for my bloods.

When I returned the following morning he took the bloods but explained I would have to wait about two weeks for the ultrasound, he had phoned the hospital and had hoped I could have been seen sooner but protocol was I had to wait! He was not impressed and I then remembered my husband has private health care through his work and I was also covered. The GP advised me to take this route to hasten things along and asked me to call him back once I had details of the scheme so he knew where to refer me. I spoke to him that afternoon and he immediately emailed my referral to a gynae consultant (at this point I thought he may be wrong and that my problem was my bowel!).

I saw the consultant at the beginning of the following week and he gave me a physical and said he thought ovarian growth/cysts and some growth in my womb but had me get an ultrasound as soon as, which was later that day in the private hospital. I then saw the consultant again on the Friday of that same week and he had the ultrasound results and the blood test results. The ultrasound had shown numerous ovarian cysts, the largest of which was 15cm in diameter. Given there was no previous history of cysts and I had no problems/symptoms they were concerned that there may be cancer or pre-cancerous cells present. The blood tests gave a low indicator of this but were not conclusive. The consultant explained that cysts of this size could rupture, bleed out or cause other problems and obviously the possibility of cancer was there too.

My family were two weeks away from a special holiday to celebrate our silver wedding, my husband's 50th and my daughter's 21st. The consultant advised against travel. I was really worried, the absence of any previous problems, my weight loss, this lump, a 15cm growth in my abdomen! I made my husband check the ultrasound report when the consultant left the room as I thought he had given the wrong info. Where could I hide a 15cm growth? I was size 10 with no protruding abdomen.

The consultant explained that both of the ovaries would be removed, it was going to be an abdominal surgery anyway due to the size of the cyst and given the chance of cancer it had to be done this way to avoid contamination. Because he was concerned about the risk of cancer he explained that his first chance at surgery was his best so in his opinion I should undergo a hysterectomy with the removal of the cervix too. The pathology tests for cancer take time and he did not want to leave anything that he may then have to remove at a later date. I had many questions and arguments but the size of the cyst really undermined my desire for laparoscopic surgery and the retention of my ovaries.

The surgery took place 10 days later, less than three weeks after my initial visit to my GP. I had a total abdominal hysterectomy, with both ovaries, tubes etc. removed. I also needed corrective surgery to my bowel, my pelvis and bladder due to adhesions caused by the large cyst; it was also fused to my uterus. The consultant did a surgical wash and also took tissue samples from other organs to test for abnormalities.

I am now five weeks on from surgery and really still trying to come to terms with it all. On the plus side my pathology results were all good and my wound is healing well (an extremely neat vertical wound considering I am very small and the cyst was very large) and I have had very little problem with pain. I have all the usual symptoms I have read about on this life-saving site – wind, sluggish bowel, struggling to come to terms with big knickers and many, many questions. Given I have no history of problems this has come as a bolt from the blue. I am now wondering about HRT, should I do it or not. My consultant wanted to wait till after the six week check. So far, I have not really experienced any symptoms, a bit warm in bed a couple of nights but then my hubby indicated he had felt warm too and the ambient temp had risen. My husband and daughter have been wonderful but I really feel all adrift with this whole situation.

The very week we should have been enjoying our wonderful family holiday, full of celebration I was shuffling about at home, popping pills, farting horribly and drinking prune juice having just been discharged from hospital. Very different from the holiday I had envisaged, sitting poolside at the wonderful villa we had chosen, enjoying the sun and sipping champagne.

Recovery Takes Time, Pauline Berry

I am three weeks post-operation today, TAH with ovaries preserved. Prior to the operation I thought I would be able to do my job, which is singing. I realized a few days ago I was nowhere near being able to do this (I was dreaming). As I can't cough or laugh without hurting whereas singing really involves all the stomach and centre of my body, it's mostly dance music too. Sadly I replaced myself for what would have been my first booking back tonight. I am settling in for the long haul of recovery which is snail slow. I am beginning to realise three weeks is very early.

The bulk of the pain is over but the twinges are nasty and change a little each day, sometimes it's like a throbbing hot needle for a couple of minutes, that was yesterday, today there is a heavy bruised feeling above the incision plus the odd string of pain which lasts just a few seconds. I hope that is normal. It's very hard to resist a nice cat stretch when I wake up in the morning. But perhaps I did that in my sleep and pulled something, feels like it.

I spend most days in bed, sleeping in the daytime sometimes too. When I first left hospital I was awake for only about four hours each day, my body seemed to need so much sleep and I feel that much sleep was really valuable and I got along the road of recovery well with that. It seems progress is slower now, three weeks in.

The swelling above the incision has a life of its own, swelling outwards much more than other times, for no apparent reason, pulling somewhat tightly on the incision when it's bigger. It changes slightly every day. The incision feels like a tight Elastoplast across my bikini line, it is pale pink though and even white in places, so no problem on the outside anyway.

I guess I just wanted to share that perhaps if expectations of quick recovery are lower; it's perhaps easier to deal with as the weeks crawl by. This six week mark to total recovery now does appear myth-like to me. I am 49 and pretty fit, but it has knocked me for six. Although I spoke to a nurse prior to find out what it would be like, the information was just 'you will be uncomfortable and it's hard to sit for any length of time in a normal chair'. This is true, but the recovery is indeed really quite debilitating as all movement I am finding is slow and restrictive. It's hard to deal with having been quite active prior.

Perhaps I am having a whinge, perhaps I have pulled a stitch inside and set myself back, I don't know. I am looking for what is 'normal' I guess.

I know I just have to wait it out – I am going a bit stir crazy (in case you can't tell).

My uterus was 22×40cms as removed during surgery. Two fibroids inside, one 10cms and one 18cms diameter, I also had several polyps. I always wondered why my tummy was so fat when I am not really a fat person.

I had lower back pain too, had been to osteopaths who only looked at the bones. When I saw the x-ray I said 'what is all that stuff next to my lower spine' and the doc thought it was just stools. I see now it was swirling fibroids. He seemed to not be aware of such possibilities. So, my lower back pain is gone, that is truly brilliant and no more massive periods causing anaemia. My whole life was based around my menstrual cycle before.

I know I have a lot to look forward to once over this recovery hump. I am interested to know about all the different little pains others' experience post-operation, and what they possibly indicate. I am hoping these new prickly little pains are a new phase of recovery and healing.

During, Yvonne's Story Continued

10th October 2007 dawned and with it was the first day I'd felt well in ages. Typical! I had to report to the hospital for midday, so we were there a little after 10am. I couldn't wait at home, and I could barely sit on the train.

There'd been a few squabbles with the insurance company over the hospital and the anaesthetist we were allowed to use, so we ended up coughing up to pay my consultant's preferred man and the insurance company worked with us to select a hospital that fitted into their pay scales and the gynaecologist's diary.

Details. Delays. I couldn't care less who inserted the needle nor which building we were in when it was inserted as long as it was done, I was asleep and all my bits were removed. It seemed dreadfully important to everyone else though.

There was another forever wait in the reception area before I was ushered to my room, but in all honesty, a delay of one minute was 'forever' in my language that day. I wasn't nervous as such, nor was I anxious. I just wanted to get to the point where the operation was in the rear view mirror and the rest of my life could begin. Hating to use a cliché, but if it involved breaking some eggs and resting for a few weeks, major surgery seemed a small price to pay for sanity and a pain free future.

The gynaecologist came by to check I was ready. With a make up free face, hair tied back and a brave smile on my face, he muttered that I looked younger than ever. I was 37½. Oddly that half seemed very important that day.

The longest walk of my life then took place. I still sometimes wake in the night, thinking about it. I had my gown on and two medical ladies (I don't know who they were) holding my arms as we walked to theatre, but we had to go at a very slow pace so my blood pressure stayed low. I was feeling amazingly well, clear headed and pain free as we ambled by the reception in the direction of the theatres. For a brief moment I thought I was going to run away. My head was screaming to stay on track, but my body was gearing up to run. I felt so sorry for what I was about to do to myself and said a little prayer.

The last thing I remember of the old me was being asked if I wanted an epidural. I said sure, I'd never had one before. He thought it would help with the pain afterwards.

I was the first in the afternoon to have my operation, which given my utter impatience was just as well. My husband settled down to watch a film in the room after we'd given each other a quick hug goodbye. He was probably more nervous than me, but then he was to be my nurse for the next 12 weeks, so I didn't blame him.

I was back in the room before I knew it. It was perhaps a couple of hours since I'd taken that slowest of walks, and other than the doziness and tubes everywhere, I was actually feeling contented. It was over. Now I had to just heal and move on. But that night I was so incredibly uncomfortable and miserable. Morphine is completely overrated; I'd clicked that stupid clicker again and again, and yet the pain was splitting me in two. Not the pain from my wound, as you'd expect, but in my spine. The epidural entry point was so painful that I really thought my spine was damaged. I was less than impressed when, in my misery, I was offered two paracetamol.

The journey home was fraught, I'll be honest. I won't go into details, but our friend picked us up and in high spirits we set off home, me sat upright. Inside of about three miles we stopped, I was in agony with flaming pain down my legs and in my back and stomach. My husband called the paramedics and, after knocking on some doors, someone kindly let me use their loo.

The lesson from that horrendous day: if you can't go home in an ambulance, then make sure you lie down on your back for the journey to avoid the downward pressure on the weak area of your body avoid liquids for a few hours prior to a journey. That bladder you had before the operation will be bruised and able to hold a thimbleful of water. It really doesn't help to take regular sips before a journey!

AFTER

They All Said I'd Never Look Back, Alison Coates

My mom, my Godmother and one of my best friends all said it was the best thing they ever did and that I would never look back. Mom was 35 when she had her hysterectomy after two children. My friend was just 41 and sadly she had not been able to have children. I was 40 when we (my consultant and I) decided to finally go with the option of a hysterectomy. I had not been married and so had not had the opportunity to have any of my own babies. It was a hard decision to make but followed five years of various kinds of hormone treatments and two laparoscopies for endometriosis. Mom had also had endometriosis.

So, an elective decision, but I was exhausted after all the hormone attempts and operations. Today a year ago I took myself off to hospital. I don't have a boyfriend so a friend came with me to the hospital and kindly held my hand and wiped away my tears while we waited for my call down to surgery. I had a full abdominal hysterectomy removing both ovaries. I nearly had a heart attack when I first saw the 13cm bikini line scar. I cried daily and was so incapacitated (in comparison to my usual sporty self) – it was such a shock. I thought I was ready for the aftermath of the op. I was so wrong.

I wanted to write this because you think you need to be brave and hold it all together, you think you can't show any weakness. Well, the first few weeks post-op will challenge you in that. It's okay. Go with it, if you need to cry then cry. I learned how to be really good at 'asking' for things.

A top tip; talk about what YOU need during the days immediately after the op. not what your friend's think you need. Friends would want to visit me after work, but by 6/7pm I was too tired for visitors, so I tried to convince them to get to me earlier. I had a nasty reaction to the pain meds and spent five days with a really upset stomach until my GP told me to stop the pain meds. I slept sitting upright because laying down set my stomach off (strangely?).

Living on my own also made the recovery somewhat challenging. I had to recruit in help to wash my long hair and had plenty of people cook me meals. I found the HA website to be very helpful and useful. I read the forum updates regularly in those early days. As you are reading this, keep reading. Someone on the forum will have had a similar operation/illness and will talk to your experience... it helps to know you are not alone.

My recovery was slow. What I also learned is we are all different. I thought that because I was fit (Triathlon, 10km swimmer, runner, cyclist) it would be a quick process – but instead of six weeks off work, it was eight. My return to work was harder than I imagined – the men in my corporate office all wanted to know if I had enjoyed my extended holiday and where had I gone. So, I also learned that I needed to be honest. It was too upsetting to 'pretend'.

I took full advantage of my work employee assistance programme one tearful day and chatted to a wonderful counsellor who gave me a bit of perspective of the reality of no longer having the choice to have babies. It's a very helpful process to talk it through with an objective person who has no vested interest in consoling me or being on my woeful, sorry side. She gave me some brilliant coping techniques and tips – practical, objective advice and highly recommended if you have the opportunity.

I started walking as soon as I could after the op, in fact the very next day. My daily five minute walks became 10 and then 20. By eight weeks I was walking for up to an hour. I believe this helped me get back into my sporting activities and also helped me clear my mind – walking was therapeutic. I had also booked a long distance swimming holiday in July so I was determined to get there healthy and ready for a beautiful time in the Mediterranean.

I started crocheting. In my second week post-op I went to a lesson (in a cab!) just to get out the house and I now have a beautiful granny blanket made up of over 100 squares. Do something with your hands; knit, sew, crochet. It's like yoga for the mind!

You are probably reading this and thinking why is she writing all of this. Well, having learned to be honest about how I was feeling, I wanted to be honest about the experience and a year on I have some perspective on this (I think). I promise you – it gets better! Today I am stronger than ever and often have to remind myself just how strong I feel. I have more energy and am less likely to snap at people. I run, swim, lift weights, walk and even did some Pilates in the early days of recovery (highly! highly! recommend).

I do sometimes get a little upset about not having children, but a very dear friend suggested to me that my natural mothering instincts need not be just for my own children. I could put those caring instincts into looking after myself for once and later into other people's children. So love yourself through the recovery and then find something you can devote your mothering instincts towards. I have nieces and nephews and plenty of friends with children. I also remember the words from the bible from Exodus which reminds us not to covet, so I try not to be jealous and try not to want what they have.

I have plenty to be happy about and grateful for in my life. I am happy, have my health back and feel amazing every day. I am early 40's and have no children, but I have SO much more. I am no longer crippled by the exhaustion this disease causes and I feel fitter than ever – I have even lost a stone in weight since the days before my op! It is possible – even on HRT.

I wanted to write this today as it's my one year anniversary of the op and I can, with conviction, now also say that 'you will never look back'. There is a reason why you have had to have the hysterectomy and all you need now do is get through the process of recovery in your own way, and time. You will see – it really will be the best decision you ever made for your health and well being. Take care and treat yourself kindly. Only you can do that.

Abdominal Radical Hysterectomy For Cervical Cancer, Amy Kinsey

Hi, I am 43 and live in South Wales. I have two children 16 and 22, a hubby and my two dogs :)

My story started late in November 2012, when I decided to make an appointment at our local surgery to have my Mirena coil changed. As

I was there and my smear was due within the next few months I decided to get it done at the same time (I hated the speculum so only doing it once seemed like a good idea). This is where my head spinning journey started.

I had the procedure done on the 19th November. Within a week I had a call from the hospital saying I had to go to the well women clinic for a colposcopy on the 29th for check-up and possible treatment for CIN3 (which meant nothing to me at the time).

Dutifully I turned up for the appointment, making sure I had a driver with me as they said that if I had treatment following the examination then it would be wise to have someone with me. So I sat in the waiting room feeling, nervous/scared/nauseous as to what to expect, I am not very good at these things at the best of times. The staff were fantastic and the gynae specialist drew me a graph showing me where I was in the CIN3/Cervical Cancer scale following the smear results. This alone was a lot to take in before having a test done, what followed was a bit more of a shock.

I laid there dreading the speculum as normal, but she was amazing. I hardly felt it at all, unlike the doctors where I nearly hit the roof in pain. She just sat there looking at the screen on my left, and said I think we had better show her what's going on with this, and not knowing what to expect, I looked at the screen, 'is that a sore patch?' I asked, looking puzzled at a small reddened square amongst a sea of whitish flesh, (an inch square at the top right of the whole screen). 'No! That's the only healthy bit.' the nurse said. With that my heart dropped and I went very quiet and apparently extremely pale. She told me they were taking a couple of biopsies, and I was left to recover and get dressed in my own time. I sat in the chair and she explained that it was not looking brilliant, and she would ring me as soon as the results were back. I went home in a daze, and my hubby was looking at me blankly not quite sure how to react.

I had a call asking if I could pop down on the 29th for a meeting about the results. With that she explained that I needed a knife cone biopsy and she was hoping to remove the CIN3 during this procedure. I was told that this had to be done before Christmas! I was immediately given the 19th December and told what to bring with me. On the day of the procedure they were fantastic, only slight cramping, but same rules, no heavy lifting and no work for weeks as I work with challenging behaviour. I was a good girl and followed the rules, hoping that was it.

Nope – I got called back in for results on the 3rd January 2013, I was told that it was cervical cancer minimum 1B1/2 but needed an MRI then and EUA the following week. My head was still spinning from the original diagnosis, so this one really knocked me off my feet. I had the tests done, and it was decided that due to a tumour higher up in the cervix, and risk of presence in glands etc., a radical hysterectomy would be on the cards and possible follow-up treatment depending on results following that.

Well I had the radical on the 4th February and the hospital was an amazing place where nothing was too much trouble and no question was stupid. I was given my own cancer specialist nurse that I could call to ask anything, and she explained the journey and how it would start. It is now coming up to three weeks, post-op, and I'm still sore and very stiff. My system still feels like it has been hit by a truck but it's to be expected as extra margins had to be taken during the operation. Glad to get the catheter and staples out and be able to move more freely. Walking round and doing extremely light chores but system still waiting to kick in and work properly. As they took everything out I now wait for the HRT side of it.

My next part of the journey will start when I get the results on the 27th February (gulp) then I will know if chemo/radiation is necessary on top of what has occurred so far. I would like to say that friends and family have been supportive, but no! They are more scared of cancer than I am and just don't know how to talk to me. I can understand this, and if you are in the same position try not to judge them too harshly for it. I am now at the cancer rage stage and am a little grumpy and bored to say the least. I am speaking to them next week about counselling and support that is available. I didn't realise just how much you need an ear to whisper into at times like this.

At the end of the day, my new motto is 'Fight Like A Girl!' And I intend getting over the RH and kicking cancers behind! I wish everyone facing a hysterectomy good luck and fast healing.

Remember – don't be afraid to ask questions– you're not alone (even if it can feel like it) – try to be positive – follow the guidelines, it hurts if you don't (smile). Hugs x

Enhanced Recovery Programme, Anita Mills

I had a prophylactic laparoscopic assisted vaginal hysterectomy with bilateral salpingo-oophorectomy on 2nd April 2012 undertaken due to strong family history of bowel and endometrial cancer. I was very apprehensive prior to admission as, at first glance, the enhanced recovery programme diary appeared to be setting out very strict guidelines.

However they were only 'guidelines'. The diary had space for comment if you weren't able to follow any instruction, i.e. sit out on day one of surgery, get dressed and eat in dining room. The staff were amazing. I had my surgery late afternoon and came back to the ward with usual catheter, IV and morphine pump. Once all tubes etc. were out the following morning, I was assisted to the en suite to wash, then to a chair. I rested on my bed when I needed to and sat out when I could.

My meals were brought to me. That may have been because I was having a trial without catheter and output needed measuring, but it appeared that the programme helps people to know what to expect and they then do the best they are able within those guidelines.

I was amazed to find that I didn't have a lot of pain or dragging sensation and in fact the worst thing was the shoulder pain resulting from the CO_2 gas dispersing! I am now five days post-op and feeling good. I realise that I was lucky that I went into surgery in good health. Good luck to anyone about to undergo similar surgery. X

It Was Like Your Soul Was Taken Away, Jenny

All started several years ago... fibroids. A wait and see approach was taken by my doctors. Eventually due to bloating, painful nauseous periods (having to take time off work), low iron count and feeling constantly tired; I decided to see a gynaecologist.

A total hysterectomy was performed on me at 51 years of age. I had wanted to keep my ovaries and discussed this with my gynaecologist and we came to an agreement – should he find anything nasty while operating he would remove them. There was nothing wrong with them ('unremarkable' was the term used in my medical report) but he took them anyway. I have since learned that even if my ovaries were left in the blood supply to them may have been hampered causing them to atrophy so who knows if it was a good or not so good thing to do.

Post-operation was a nightmare. Two weeks after I went into full menopause, dreadful sweats, hot flushes (several an hour!), headaches, foggy head, balance problems. I toughed it all out without medication (I tried over the counter products to no avail).

A complication caused by the actual operation (keyhole) has been peripheral nerve damage to my upper left thigh which manifests as slight numbness to the touch and occasionally a little weakness – I am only vaguely aware of it now.

Five months on I feel better especially in the lower back tummy region, have more energy but the head feelings are still a bother... better if I get good sleeps.

Some nights I have had to resort to a sleeping tablet as symptoms have overwhelmed me but I take each day as it comes and pay more attention to my emotional and physical needs.

I am a bit of a nervous nelly and had post-natal depression with my first son (24 years ago but not with my other two sons). These symptoms have returned but as I recognise them for what they are (hormonally induced) I can cope better now.

Overall menopause for me (surgically induced) has meant like a kind of death but with sites like the HA (which have helped tremendously in verbalising how we all feel) and mentoring with friends, there is life on the other side of it and I can see it as a renewal or perhaps a stock-take of how to move forward.

I was completely naive about the menopause and it was like my first period and having my first baby – shocking... but I have gotten used to it like all great changes in our female life!

Thank you so much for all the information you have provided and to all the women that have shared their experiences.

There are many experiences involved with a hysterectomy and it really comes down to the individual woman herself and also our general health.

Five years on I am still having daily hot flushes but not as intense (which still continue to wake me up especially here in Sydney in the summer).

Stress plays a part so I have to slow down and pace myself more and often have naps when I can – I still work four days (20 hours) a week but can't do any more than that as the job is in a hospital medical record dept. and is quite heavy work at times.

With aging in general (I am now 57) it is sometimes hard to know, for me that is, if I would have got all the ghastly symptoms had I gone into menopause naturally.

I feel that because I was still having a regular period at 51 the surgical hysterectomy threw me into instant menopause and consequently many horrid symptoms as it does for most women prior to the 'change'.

When I look back perhaps I should have gone onto HRT but with all the scare mongering at the time I avoided it like the plague! I did try remedies but nothing seems to work except improving my diet and exercise. Forums online were a life line as we could all compare the array of symptoms we were all having which helped tremendously from going completely crazy with fear!

To be honest women whom I had known and had taken HRT were back to square one with hot flushes and typical menopausal symptoms when they went off their HRT. So, I avoided the hormones because of this, maybe to my detriment as I feel rather worn out by it all.

You have asked for a story on my hysterectomy – all I can say is that hindsight is always a wonderful thing. Had I had my time over again I would seek out another opinion and also medical procedures that could remove fibroids without the total removal of my uterus and ovaries. I let myself be talked into a hysterectomy and bilateral salpingo-oophorectomy without really understanding the ramifications. Also, I don't think the medics (who are male normally) really understand the gravity of taking the female reproductive system out (for non life threatening diseases).

My GP said something which I will always remember. His mother had had a hysterectomy and she had said to him it was like your soul had been taken – which I am inclined to agree with (she was also getting a few hot flushes into her 70's!!).

This all sounds like doom and gloom but what keeps me going is that I could have been hit by a bus on the way out of the hospital! I try to keep things in perspective. There are so many people who are much worse off than me who have terribly difficult medical problems to deal with on a daily basis.

Six Years On, Carole

I remember waking up the day after the operation thinking – I have made it through the night, it doesn't feel too bad and it can only get better. Who was I kidding? No amount of reading or talking had prepared me for the sense of vulnerability I felt as I left the hospital, or over the following weeks.

That first journey from the hospital ward to the main entrance was long and frightening – I remember people getting out of the lift I had just passed making a lot of noise and sounding boisterous – would they bump into me? I couldn't see them, I felt scared and tears started to well up inside. I was used to feeling physically strong and fit and now I felt weak and unable to resist anything.

Having my mobile phone with me became very important in the following weeks as I slowly began to walk further and further outside – it made me feel safer.

I religiously stuck to the hospital exercise walking routine and initially all was going well but by week four I was struggling and in pain – I was pushing too hard too soon, for me. It knocked my confidence and my progress. I was clearly going to have to learn to be patient.

As hard as I tried to 'do the right thing' to help me get better it wasn't happening and I felt a growing concern that I was falling behind. I know now that is illogical as we are all different but I was so used to being able to be a key player in 'actively' making myself better at times of illnesses and for the first time I just seemed to be getting it wrong.

Being alone and unemployed didn't help as I felt under pressure (from myself) to get better quickly so I could start working again but without the option of a phased introduction to work I had to be confident I could make the grade.

By three months I still hadn't had a full night's sleep (due to backache) and was still experiencing discomfort in my stomach area. I wasn't feeling confident and I was feeling increasingly frustrated and tearful. In the end it was several trips to my osteopath that did the trick and helped me turn the corner. By releasing all the tension in my pelvis (I'd gone into and become stuck in protective mode) I was finally able to sleep on my sides and stride out in my walks. It was around this time I also stopped religiously doing the exercises I had been given by the hospital – it was time to just relax and let my body do it's own thing and stop 'over trying' to get better too soon. My activity levels began to increase, my levels of frustration dropped and I finally began to regain some of my old levels of confidence. Now to find that job.

Six years on: It is hard to look back to a time that seems so long ago now. That first year or so was an emotional time for me. The feelings of physical vulnerability had made me begin to think of my old age and how that might be, as well as coming to terms with the fact that some options in life were over, led to quite a bit of re-evaluation of life so far and what the future held.

I found a job about eight months after the operation – it was only four days a week to start with but I wasn't too disappointed – it gave me more time to explore new interests and do a bit of nurturing. I remember still being a bit cautious of my body for some time, worrying if that tweak or bump was something to worry about – my doctor reassured me that this was just some scar tissue and it may take a year to settle down completely (which it did). It is difficult to say at what point I no longer thought about the operation but I am now employed full time, happy, healthy and really appreciate the freedom the operation has given me.

A Difficult Pregnancy Led To My Hysterectomy, Claire Reeves

I became pregnant with my third child in September 2003 and I was 40. Our delight soon turned to concern when I was told I had placenta praevia grade IV and would not have a natural birth as I'd had before. I would have to have a c-section as my placenta had implanted right at my cervix. They had hoped it would grow up and move but it didn't. Worse still I was told I must go into hospital two months before I was due in case of a serious bleed. So I spent eight weeks sitting in hospital waiting for the c-section which I was dreading.

The day arrived and I was first up at 8am. General anaesthetic and eight hours later I was still in recovery as I was continually bleeding and losing a lot of blood. Eventually they got it to stop but I was very unwell. A few days later I went home but my time there had completely traumatised me – not only for the length I had been in hospital but the stressful birth.

Then started a period for four years! Yes, I bled continually for four years, I had all kinds of treatment, procedures, medication, everything but it wouldn't stop. It was then my consultant said I had to have a full hysterectomy.

So the following week I had my op, but bearing in mind my trauma the last time I had been in hospital I was a complete nervous wreck.

The nurses were very kind, but in my head it was complete terror. It ended up in me not being about to be anesthetised in a gentle way!! But anyway I would have got up and run off if I hadn't had the silly gown on!

Woke up in HDU where I had great care from the nurses but was very unwell as the general anaesthetic made me very sick. Two days later and I was still being sick – but was feeling much better.

A week later and I was home and recovering slowly. It took a while to feel better physically but four years on and I believe it was the right thing. I started on HRT but eventually came off it. The thing with having a hysterectomy is you sort of crash straight into menopause not the gradual, natural one like most ladies. Hot flushes are a pain but manageable. I'd recommend this op to anyone even though I had a difficult time – looking back it was the right thing to do.

That Lady With A Cervix, Sally

At the age of 42, the pain and heavy periods were escalating each month.

Then I started bleeding after sex. I was concerned that I had cancer. It was only at this stage that I went to the doctors.

I was shocked when the doctor ensured that I had an ultrasound scan within two weeks. The lady who did the internal scan started putting red crosses on her screen; I asked if it was cancer. She said it was not sinister, but looked like adenomyosis. I had not heard of that before, I asked if it was curable. 'It depends on your attitude to surgery' was her reply.

I was terrified of what I had. The internet was fantastic, and explained that it was like endometriosis, but in the womb muscle. The only real cure was a hysterectomy. But I had a terrible memory of my emergency caesarean, which had left me traumatised, and with only one child, as I was too afraid to risk giving birth again.

I refused to have the operation, but eight months later I was unable to get to work, or leave the house for the first few days of each period, and then I passed out from the cramps at work.

So I agreed to the operation, but I felt I was on a conveyer belt. No consultation, just a date and turn up. I had no idea how long my stay would be, or what to expect. I cancelled two dates, but knew that I had to have it done. So I saw my doctor again, who confirmed it was the only way. I then arranged with the hospital to see the ward, and spoke to the sister, she was very helpful, explained about pain relief and the length of stay.

On the internet I had read about a sub total hysterectomy. The internet had become my knowledge. I decided that's what I would have; keep my ovaries, and my cervix, only take out the thing causing the pain. But there was nobody to explain my decision to.

The day of the operation, I refused to sign the consent form; they wanted to take the lot. Two hours before the operation a young male doctor came, and I had to explain why I wanted to keep my cervix. So in very detailed words I described how I didn't feel that I would be complete if it wasn't there, he looked shocked. Next I had about eight doctors and staff around me, to explain it all again, it felt that I wasn't allowed to be a person, with emotions, only a number to process.

Eventually the surgeon agreed. So I had what I wanted, but everybody knew my reasons. That was a year ago, and I am pleased that I made a stand. My doctor calls me 'that lady with a cervix'. Sex isn't quite like it used to be, but I can feel my cervix contract, and still feel like a woman.

Meniere's Disease Linked To Monthly Cycle, Debi Wilson

I am a 46 years old female and I am profoundly deaf with good speech and I was having on-going dizzy spells and was usually always worse around the time of my cycle which was around 21st to 30th of the month.

I was having on-going appointments at the audiology department and seeing consultants at the ear, throat and eye clinic. This went on for two years with vertigo, fluid retention, vomiting severe motion sickness and I was virtually incapable of everyday daily tasks with on-going memory loss and finally I was diagnosed with this blasted Meniere's disease.

However this Meniere's disease was getting worse and worse that it was affecting my life at work and socially, so I started to look at my pattern of eating with the food so I changed my diet reducing salt and caffeine and chocolate etc. This did help to a certain extent but by the 21st to 31st of the month I was affected tremendously and my quality of life was taken from me until one night, through the night I was awoken from my sleep with blood on my bed sheets.

I had actually started my period and the room was spinning with the furniture round and round, and if I moved my head it made the spinning sensation worse with increased pressure in the ear. You almost feel you have been drugged and have no control of yourself in trying to stop this vertigo. It takes over your life and can leave you so shattered that you sleep for several hours.

The other side effects I had were double vision, lack of coordination, sweating, hearing loss and sometimes tinnitus.

So, on the next follow-up appointment at the ENT Dept. to see the consultant I asked him. 'Why is it that I have a Meniere attack when I am menstruating?'

The consultant was baffled so then he referred me to a gynaecologist who took blood tests. I was injected in the abdomen every month with a drug called Zoladex which prevents you from having a cycle every month. This finally worked, I had no more brainfog days; I was vertigo free; I was feeling normal, alert and I got my quality life back so I proceeded with this drug for 18 months. The consultant decided it was linked to my monthly cycle and was only advisable to be taken for no more than six months.

I went to see a private gynaecologist who insisted that my hormones were making me very ill and it was a rare case of Meniere's disease linked to a menstrual cycle. He decided not to allow my natural period back after 18 months and decided to offer me a radical total abdominal hysterectomy and bilateral salpingo-oophorectomy to completely obliterate my menstrual cycle.

And now I am symptom free, but I do still have on-going dizzy spells during 21st to 30th of the month. They aren't as severe as the Meniere's disease attacks where I would have been dysfunctional and incapacitated for three weeks of the month with the symptoms, and now it would be just nine days of the month.

I guess I have to thank my GP, my consultant and gynaecologist for giving me back my quality of life.

What A Gift Having My Hysterectomy, Deva Shore

I was born with these diseases and suffered for many years with polycystic ovaries and endometriosis. I am now 58 and in our day you were virtually classed as a hypochondriac and ignored. Fortunately things have changed as my 29 year old daughter has both these diseases now.

I have to say having a total hysterectomy, ovaries and all at 34 was a blessing. I definitely don't miss having a period and all the pain that went with it. I am thankful to my doctor for listening and discovering my condition and am blessed to have three beautiful daughters.

All Over Now, Diane Mann

Hi, I had my hysterectomy in October 2012, they removed my womb and ovaries and the surrounding tissue but left my cervix. The op went well with no problems.

I was on a morphine pump, which I didn't use that much. Moving was very sore to start with but did improve and I left hospital five days later.

At home things continued to be fine with no loss down below, I am just very tired. A week later I got an infection in my wound which cleared with antibiotics. Moving got easier and I started to do little things.

At six weeks I had a hospital appointment which I thought would be okay, just a check-up and go away to enjoy your life; but no, I was told they found pre-cancerous cells in my womb so I would have to have another op to the remove cervix. I was a mess but with the support of my partner came to terms with it.

I had my cervix removed in March 2013 by keyhole surgery and everything is going well. I received a call from hospital a week later to be told everything was clear, nothing had spread.

I'm now going to focus on getting back to normal and having pain free months with no bleeding. I have suffered from some menopausal symptoms but am coping so far. I just want to say that I was terrified of having my bits removed but it was the best choice I made and the end result is worth it, just be brave take it slowly and you will get there in the end.

A letter to My Dear Beautiful Body Parts, Dierdra Tara Michelle

So much of the focus of the past few months has been on you and what is the best for the whole 'nation of me' in regards to our present situation. I am so sorry that the invasion of 'growth gone wild' has made your existence difficult and brought pain to us all. I am very glad that we are entering an action that will take away the pain and help to ensure many more years of life as a whole. Well…sort of as a whole.

I do regret that this assurance comes with the sacrifice of you, my beloved Uterus and Cervix. I completely honour the sacrifice that you are making to bring wellness to the whole. I know that this will surely mean the death of you and am beyond words for the choice of that sacrifice.

I do not know what life will be without you, for you have been a big part of me since the beginning of my life. I have placed so much of my sexual identity, both good and bad, upon your shoulders.

I regret how foolishly I have allowed the harmful actions of others, actions resulting as emotional responses within me, to focus on you and my surrounding sexual organs. I know that I have never allowed you to be fully and completely all you could be. I held you back because of my fear that the abusers violently inserted into my life. In turn, I acknowledge that I channelled that abuse into you as a way to hide the pain. For this I apologise.

I am sad that our journey together did not go another way and that I never truly learned to bask in the beauty of the sexuality that you were part of within me. You know I always vacillated between thinking myself as not enough sexually and hating that I had a sexuality that so often brought others to hurt me. In those brief moments when I could break through those lies, I could see how beautifully you embraced life and the experiences we were given. I hold you in awe for this. Thank You! Please set within my spirit the ability to live in those breakthrough moments from this day forward. I ask this as an honour to your sacrifice.

You both were so instrumental in helping the lives that came through me into being. I cannot express enough gratitude to you for this. I adore the interactions that those children have brought and all they offer to the world, the future, and unto me. You cradled them in the most secret parts of their construction and their life would not be without your efforts. Your greatest offering to life is this task of allowing our small conjoining of cells to become an independent life, which is completely self-sustaining as a whole being when you finish your task. Every mammalian life that moves upon this earth has a uterus and cervix like you to thank. Thank you for your part in this as a way to ensure the existence of life, as we know it!

I offer my gratitude tonight with this ceremony of fire and blood to you. Gratitude for all you brought to the world throughout the existence of life. Gratitude for all you brought to me through the creation of children. Gratitude for all you brought to me through sexual pleasures and the union that it creates with lovers. Gratitude for the sacrifice you are making tomorrow to ensure my life into the future. I offer up Gratitude in advance for the success of that surgery that we will be part of together. I offer you Gratitude, Gratitude and more Gratitude. I thank you and love you and wish you great rest from this day forwards. Rest in Peace my friends. With Gratitude, Love and Happiness.

I Did Not Want To Have This Op But Had To, Elena Micallef-Borg

For many years, I was told to have a hysterectomy but did not want to. Firstly I had miscarried and never had any children and was hoping to have one; and secondly simply because I was so scared. I was also completely not ready for this op as for me hysterectomy spells old age which I did not feel was for me!

The 25th November 2011, arrived and I had my operation, I was so afraid that I would not be able to cope with the pain, but thank God I managed. I had three massive fibroids, each 10cm x 10cm, my uterus was that of a 26 week gestation, they were pressing on my kidneys and bladder, and I ended up having an up and down incision.

On the whole I cannot complain about my recovery, I had terrible flushes and therefore started having HRT in January 2012. They have lessened but still get the occasional flush here and there! Oh well, I guess I just have to carry a hand fan wherever I go!

The only two things that really bother me are my interrupted sleep – I used to manage sleeping a whole eight hours with no problem at all. Since my op, I get up at least three times and I am really tired; and the obvious other is weight gain. In January 2012, I joined a gym and was using the treadmill, watching what I eat and still put on weight. I just suggest that you seek help with a real nutritionist if necessary. Don't go for faddy diets excluding certain foods, we need to eat everything!

Prior to my operation, I also took vitamins which I believe helped me with the operation and recovery, and basically that was Vitamin C, Vitamin E, fish oils and turmeric. Another tip which I would like to share is take charcoal tablets after your first meal after the operation and add olive oil. I managed to go to the bathroom with no pain whatsoever and get rid of all the unwanted wind which is so painful.

I do feel more tired than before my op but I think I am getting better. I hope that all you women who have to do this op will find my story of help; I was really petrified before my op, because I thought that I would not cope with the pain but I did. I was afraid that I would have complications with the stitches because normally a simple scratch would turn septic, but I managed!

I just take one day at a time and try to be as positive as possible! Sometimes I managed, sometimes I fail and sometimes I laugh! But I am just thankful to God that I am healthy and I think that is the most important thing to remember!

A New Beginning At 25, Elizabeth Stable

At the age of 25 I had to make probably the biggest decision of my life. I started my period when I was 10, and right from the very beginning they were a nightmare, I was off school every time it came because they were so heavy they used to come through onto the seats. I was also in so much pain, I remember my mum took me to the doctors and they said there was nothing they could do for me as I was so young.

At the age of 14 they put me onto the pill to see if it would help to control them. It didn't. I used to have to wear three pairs of knickers and six pads and it would still come through onto my trousers and onto the seats at school, I was so embarrassed.

I had terrible mood swings; I was a nightmare to live with. I met my husband and we began to try for a family, after two and half years of trying they did some blood tests and found out I wasn't ovulating every month.

I was sent to see a fertility specialist who wanted to do a laparoscopic investigation, however a week before I was meant to go in I found out I was pregnant, I was overjoyed as they had told me it would be very difficult for me to fall pregnant. However it wasn't to be and a week later I lost my baby, thankfully I went on to have three beautiful babies, two boys and a girl, although I also lost a further two babies.

I bled all through my pregnancies which, as you can imagine, was very distressing. The doctors said that pregnancy should sort my periods out and make them regular and less heavy. A few months after my second son was born they did a vaginal exam and saw that I had very bad erosion on my cervix. I went in for an operation to fix this and they thought after that the bleeding would be controlled again.

After my daughter was born and I had my first period it didn't go away for two months then after that I would bleed three out of every four weeks. I decided to get sterilised in the hope it would help me, I knew I didn't want any more children so if it was going to help then I was all for it, but yet again it didn't.

I tried the pill again and the coil, nothing worked! They then put me onto monthly injections of Decapeptyl which basically stopped my ovaries releasing an egg therefore stopping my periods. I was 24 when this happened; it was the first time in 14 years I had had a break from the pain and the constant bleeding. Although the mood swings stayed, my periods stopped and I felt I had my life back. However, because the injections I was getting took a little bit of my bone density every time I got one I was only allowed six so my joy was short lived.

I spoke to my consultant who decided that it would be a good idea to try microwave ablation which could give me up to five years of very light or no periods, although it meant another operation. I was all for it if it would give me a break – 'Bring it on!' I said.

So the day came for me to have the MA done. I went to theatre and was told that it would take about an hour, however when I came round it had only been 30 minutes and I knew something was wrong. The doctor came to see me and told me they had extreme difficulty in dilating my cervix and because of this they had perforated my womb and had to stop the operation immediately. I was devastated; this was my chance of having a few years break.

I'd had enough and I asked for a hysterectomy, I couldn't take it anymore, the mood swings were getting worse I would shout at my husband for little things, like not putting the shopping away the right way, or the kids would be shouted at for nothing. I asked my doctor for a hysterectomy, he said he wouldn't do it on someone as young as me; he wanted to try the microwave ablation again only laparoscopic this time, although he couldn't give me a definite answer as to whether there was a chance it would happen again.

So after talking it through with my husband I decided to get a second opinion. My GP referred me to a consultant who listened to what I had been through in my own words instead of reading my notes; he understood that I wanted no more children. He told me that really a hysterectomy was the only medical option for me as I had really tried everything. He agreed to do it for me. I was so overjoyed words can't explain.

I was set to go in on the 21st September 2011. The gynaecologist came to see me and explained to me that he would perform a vaginal hysterectomy, leaving my ovaries behind but taking my womb and cervix. I was very nervous but also excited at the same time. I was wheeled into theatre went to sleep, woke up a few hours later and it was done. I wasn't in any pain because of the pain killers and I had a catheter in and also a vaginal pack.

My husband and son came to see me that night but it's just a blur, I think I slept through most of the time they were there. It had hit my oldest son the hardest, he hated to see me in hospital; when I had the microwave ablation I was supposed to be in and out, but I was in for five days, he came to the hospital expecting to take me home but his dad had to explain to him I couldn't get home – he cried his heart out which is why I decided I couldn't do it anymore.

The next day it was time to get my catheter removed and the vaginal pack. I really wasn't looking forward to this, the nurse said that I would feel pressure when my pack was removed, well her words were you will probably feel like your insides are falling out, didn't help the nerves. When she was removing the pack I just kept thinking how much has he put in there? It just kept coming and coming.

That night they were having a problem with my blood pressure it was very low because of the pain killers so the monitor was continually beeping and the nurses had me laying this way and that way. The next day I had to have a bladder scan because my bladder wasn't emptying as it should be. I was told to drink plenty of water to get it working again. My gynaecologist came to see me and told me that I was allowed to go home the next day; he also said that my womb had been sent to the lab and I would get the results in about four weeks.

Of course hearing that I started to assume all sorts of things had been found. Google really isn't a good place to look up womb and lab. My ovaries went into shock for a few weeks, which was tough. My sleeping pattern was terrible – sleeping all day up all night, the hot flushes were constant and I was worried that they had gone into shock permanently; however they got better each day. Before I knew it I was four weeks post-op and I had begun to walk a wee bit, which after being stuck in the house with nothing but day time TV and gossip magazines was great. My family had been my support line.

I am now just over a year post-op, and I have to say it was the best decision I have ever made, sure there were days before I had it when I would sit and cry and say to my husband I wouldn't be a proper woman, and what if something went wrong with the operation. I think everyone has fears, especially when they are young. I wanted to share my story just to show that even though I was very young, at only 25, I know I made the right decision.

I am now pain and period free and I have my life back, me and my husband renewed our wedding vows on September 29th, a year and a week after I had my op, I have my life back now and this is just the beginning.

My Hysterectomy Story, Hazel Gee

When you read my story about my hysterectomy I am sure that most of you will think me a very stupid woman, because I buried my head in the sand you see, to the symptoms of cancer of the womb, of endometrial cancer. In the end I had to go the doctor about the bleeding that had been going on sporadically for almost a year. I know why I didn't go for so long; it was partly embarrassment and partly the nagging fear of what they would find. From the time I went to the doctor and was referred for an ultrasound scan which led to a hysteroscopy, a clinic visit for the findings of the hysteroscopy and my op was less than two months.

When I went for the results of the hysteroscopy I was told that I had cancer and it would require a hysterectomy, with removal of my ovaries and tubes, a procedure that goes under the baffling label of 'total abdominal hysterectomy and bilateral salpingo-oophorectomy'. In layman's language this is the removal of the uterus, both fallopian tubes and both ovaries via an abdominal incision and basically it is the removal of all baby-making apparatus. At 62 this was not an issue but my heart goes out to anyone of childbearing age that receives this news. I wasn't totally shocked; it was just my worst fears being confirmed.

The consultant I saw that day was wonderful; he sat there calmly as I almost held out an imaginary diary trying to see when I would be able to fit the op in. He gave me a long look and I sensed that the op wouldn't wait for me to decide the date and I said to him, 'You're talking sooner rather than later aren't you?' He nodded, looking glad to have me focused and he went on to explain that the womb is a bag and that the cancer is within the bag (womb) so by removing the bag intact I had a good chance of a complete recovery.

I will be honest here that I felt sort of annoyed that I had cancer. I was then taken to another room by the Macmillan nurse who was present when I had been told the news. In the room she was saying things to me, giving me leaflets on cancer, I felt like I was losing control and inwardly directed my resentment of that towards her. I felt like the cancer was nudging in on my independence and that I was getting a taste of what was to come.

The leaflets continued when I attended another hospital for my pre-op assessment. The waiting room's tables in the oncology clinic were strewn with information on cancer, a notice board held more. I felt that resentment again, I knew that I had cancer but I didn't want it staring me in the face that way. Once in the clinic and being assessed yet more literature was handed to me. I felt overwhelmed by it. I felt that I had stepped into some sort of game that everyone else knew the rules of and I was the new girl. It was like a well-oiled machine, the pre-op assessment clinic. I was turned out the other end, blood tested, chest X-rayed, MRSA test swabbed and counselled re the risks and still reeling with the news that the op date was less than a week away. I went home with John to resume my mission of filling the freezer with good, home cooked food.

I had kept the whole thing from my grown up children. It was hard, not knowing how things would turn out but the kids kept me going; just carrying on as normal all through that Christmas of 2009 was bitter sweet. As we took the decorations down I was more methodical than usual I bought some storage crates in case I wasn't there the next year, making it easier for the following Christmas.

In January 2010 not long before the op I went to my grandkid's birthday party; that was very difficult. I gave my eldest daughter an 18th birthday banner for her eldest daughter's 18th 'in case I couldn't get to her birthday' in early February, knowing full well I wouldn't as it would be days after my op. I wrote letters, to be either given or sent as emails to our kids just before the op, I hope reassuring them. Once they knew I felt relieved, I suddenly felt stronger as the secrecy had been draining but had got me through, giving a sense of normality. I work freelance and at that time had several students on my books receiving my dyslexia support. I gave them the option of switching to another tutor; none took me up on the option and I subsequently saw them through to attain their GCSEs and others graduate at their respective degree, Masters and PhD levels.

Back in my pre-op world I cooked for the freezer bagging it up in portion sizes. It felt a bit like the nesting process you go through when about to give birth, a little part of me wondered if I instinctively knew that I was going to die but not once did I give in to self-pity and that gave me strength. I don't like to hear folk talk incessantly about their conditions, hospital; appointments and blood tests etc. as if they have no other life outside of this.

It was a very cold January in 2010, I couldn't seem to be able to get warm, and I don't know if this was due to the cancer. Combined, the tumour and the fibroid that they had discovered at the same time were the size of a four month pregnancy. I think it's strange that they compare cancer to a pregnancy because with a pregnancy you have something to hold and to love, assuming all goes well you have a baby that you take home to nurture and protect. I suppose it is something that a woman can grasp the size of; they could hardly say you have a tumour the size of a potato, an orange or a plum for example because these could come from the fruit and veg section of Waitrose or be Tesco everyday and size could vary considerably.

1st February 2010, the day of the op dawned and as we travelled along the coast road at 6am the moonlight shone on the water as first light broke it was a beautiful sight. It was a long, long day as there were several emergencies, which quite rightly took precedence, and it was teatime by the time I went to theatre. I hadn't eaten or drunk since the night before and my head was thumping with I guess dehydration. From early morning I watched others being taken and brought back zonked out and wished that it was me (I observed that dyed black hair is not a good look on a white-faced older woman fresh back from theatre)! It felt bizarre sat on the trolley in an ante room and being given a mag to read as the theatre sister chatted and folded and sorted sterile gowns for theatre packs as if she had just brought the washing in off the line and I'd called in for a chat.

I felt incredibly calm as I was wheeled in and was sent off to sleep. I wasn't uncomfortable when I woke up. Back on the ward I received excellent care all through that first night. It was the following days as the morphine drip was removed that the pain kicked in but a cocktail of medication meant it was never unbearable.

Going out of the ward to the toilet the first time I swore with the pain...a lot...and later apologised to my ward mates. It felt like climbing Everest; overcoming the pain when moving around, going to the toilet, having a shower and doing the most basic things like getting in and out of bed. I had requested no sweets and chocolate to be brought in as I wanted to give my body the very best chance of healing and recovery. I took packs of little pots of fruit in fruit juice in; there are plenty in the supermarkets to choose from. I drank a lot of water in the theory that it would flush out the anaesthetic, I don't know if I was talking out of my backside thinking that but I do know that I did very well regarding getting over the anaesthetic and resuming eating small meals and drinking without nausea. By the time I was ready for home five days later I was moving around a lot better but had a long way to go – and I was very grateful for all that they had done for me.

I hated not being able to do stuff post-op. I needed help to do the most basic jobs but my stubborn, determined, independent nature helped me on the road to a good recovery. It is no good lying around indefinitely post-op. Some activity little and often, good snooze breaks, a bit of telly in the day, a sensible balance worked for me and as a relatively old codger (62 when I had the op) I think I did okay. If you are determined to move on after the op and after cancer you will succeed. I resumed seeing students less than two weeks post-op – something that would have been impossible if I worked outside the home. I am not/was not superwoman I was on pain killers but there was nothing wrong with my brain and I feel the resuming of as normal a life as possible post-op was good for me. I had been an idiot and worried about the bleeding and been scared to get it investigated for too long – I wanted to just get on with my life.

I am now three years on and have just been discharged from the oncology clinic. I planted sweet peas today; I remember planting some when I was first recovering and it was such a difficult task and I needed help but I did it. Our eight grandchildren are all growing up fast; they are my moon and my stars and have given me such extra special pleasure since the op.

To anyone having gloomy thoughts about an impending op or maybe you are post-surgery I say to you, stop looking back and look forward. It's your womb (and maybe other lady bits) you are going to lose/have lost not your life. I am so very lucky and so very grateful. I am grateful to the fates for my extra years; I am grateful for the surgeon and anaesthetist and all involved in theatre that day for ridding me of cancer. I am grateful for the nurses for their humour and loving care. I am grateful for the Macmillan's as I grew to not only trust them but to recognise the breadth of their role in cancer care. I always thought that they were for the dying, dying of cancer. The Macmillan's attached to the hospital have always been at the end of the phone for me once home and I soon came to realise how vital they are in cancer care. My needs have been purely practical like discussing matters that I would rather talk to them about with post-op issues as they have the first-hand experience rather than bothering my doctor. They are warm, friendly, approachable and so knowledgeable.

I did get to read some of those leaflets eventually. In the main there is a need for most gynae oncology leaflets to be condensed into one booklet for those that don't have the internet at home. It would be a good option to give patients a choice of how they access the information if they do have internet access; maybe a card showing the website that would fit in their purse so they could go online and access the information or perhaps the website for the information could go on their appointment card, saving paper, ink and printing costs. We did eventually get through the casseroles that I had cooked for the freezer – they were a godsend actually!

My final gratitude has to go to my slave, my husband, that fetched and carried for me when I was in early recovery, it wasn't easy for me to ask for and accept help but I had no choice, as independent as I am there were some tasks that I just couldn't do early on.

I would say it was 12 months before it dawned on me I no longer felt 'post-op'. And now that I am discharged from oncology I await a clinic appointment for an anterior wall prolapse, this was found at my final check-up. It is very different feeling to when I was waiting for surgery for cancer with all the uncertainty that filled my head at that time. The experience will no doubt be another tale to tell. Good wishes to all readers!

Go For It, Anne

I had my two children, both boys, at aged 38 and 40, suffering a cervical prolapse temporarily after each. After a few months with plenty of pelvic floor exercises, the symptoms went away, until a relapse a some years later due to stress, I think. Again, a period of exercising did the trick and I was prolapse-free for another few years. Then in 2005 the prolapse returned. Now aged 52 nothing was going to make it go away this time.

I ended up with an emergency admission to hospital one year later having become convinced I had absorbed the tampon I was using as a sort of pessary!

I was referred to the gynae clinic and fitted with a proper pessary, discussed the matter with the consultant and despite always vowing I would not have a hysterectomy for what I regarded as a minor complaint, was convinced by him it was the best course of action. My mother, auntie and grandmother (maternal) had had the same condition and remedy. The consultant explained it was possible the condition would return if I just had a pelvic floor repair and that the operation with vaginal hysterectomy would not be significantly more complicated. I read the literature provided by the association and decided it was the best way forward.

How glad I am that I did! Just before my op it was found I was severely anaemic (6.7) and needed a blood transfusion. I knew I was a bit anaemic (pale gums) and was taking a vitamin with iron supplement, but had no other symptoms. It turned out I had fibroids (again, no symptoms) and this may have been causing the anaemia. Other tests have proved negative and iron levels are now getting back to normal. Also, I had suffered back pain for many years. This has completely gone since the hysterectomy (in fact it immediately disappeared). The consultant had been careful to say he could not promise this would happen and my GP thought it was muscle spasm. Naturally, I am over the moon.

Finally during the operation they found an ovarian cyst and my left ovary was removed. So I have effectively had four conditions cured by one operation!

The worst part of the op (I had a spinal anaesthetic but with complete sedation) was the pain after the spinal wore off – not being able to get the combination of pain killers quite right at first, but this only lasted one day and night. Also, I was not being able to wee straight away when the catheter was removed. Eventually a little running of the tap did the trick!

My stitches (rear passage repair) were very sore and tender for a few days on returning home, very much like stitches after childbirth, but within a few days this problem also disappeared.

I had one or two times of feeling shaky in hospital with a feeling of slight depression, I think due to the shock to the system of the operation, but this has cleared up.

I am now nearly three months on I have plenty of energy as long as I don't overdo it and I am looking forward to returning to work in the near future. To anyone who is considering hysterectomy for prolapse I would say, GO FOR IT!

Post Script further investigations revealed I have coeliac disease. This was diagnosed four months after the hysterectomy, and it was the coeliac disease which was the cause of the anaemia – only temporarily treated by a blood transfusion. It seems likely that the anaemia was the cause of the recurring prolapse.

With hindsight, it should have been investigated before the hysterectomy took place. However I don't regret having the hysterectomy as it revealed I had fibroids and an ovarian cyst. I have much more energy now the coeliac has been diagnosed and treated with a gluten-free diet. I believe this undiagnosed coeliac disease was the cause of my previous miscarriages. Coeliac disease has many symptoms, one of which is severe anaemia caused by damage to the gut lining preventing it from absorbing nutrients properly.

My Life Began At 43, Janice Wynne

Ever since I first started my periods at the age of 12 I never really dealt with them very well. When I was pregnant with my first child in 1987 I found I had anaemia which is why I always used to suffer with heavy periods. I was put on iron which I took for many years.

It wasn't until about a year ago I went to my doctor feeling washed out, had a blood test and found I had hardly any iron in me. Hysterectomy was my only option. I had my op in June 2012, was on pain killers for about three weeks and then from seven weeks no more bleeding.

I have my life back, I can plan things weeks ahead without worrying if I am going to be okay. I may not have thought it at the time of recovery but it's the best thing I ever did.

My Womb Cancer Journey, Jennie Bennett

I have a feeling the story of my womb cancer journey may turn into War and Peace but I also hope that it will be quite cathartic and help to banish a few of my demons along the way. I was going to keep this short, but my womb cancer journey has been a long and at times painful one. I am going to give my account warts and all about how having womb cancer has affected me both physically and mentally. This could get messy!

For as long as I can remember I had had problems with my periods which started when I was eleven years old, I felt this was quite barbaric for a child who was still wearing vests! My periods would be all or nothing; I wouldn't have a period for months, then I would bleed very heavily for months. I was quite often sent home from secondary school and have vivid memories of sitting at the back of the bus crying with the crippling pain. I would flood without warning and it really started to affect my quality of life. I was constantly going backwards and forwards to the doctors and being referred to and discharged from the gynaecology consultant.

One morning when I was in my mid twenties I woke up in so much pain I thought I was about to give birth; I thought I was going to be one of the ladies you see on TV shows, 'I didn't know I was pregnant'! The pain was excruciating and for four days I went backwards and forwards to the doctors but I was told I was just constipated! By the end of the fourth day I was at the end of my tether. I asked my dad to take me to the GP out of hours. I was immediately admitted to hospital where I was put on morphine and stayed for five days with a ruptured ovarian cyst. I thought I had also developed Tourette's syndrome at this point as every time I moved I felt like I was being stabbed and swore with the pain!

I put on a lot of weight when I was in my early 20s and I felt like I was treated almost like a drug addict by health professionals because of this; I was described as 'stout' by my gynaecologist who did very little to help me following a failed laparoscopy as 'I was too fat'. I was totally mortified but was still stuck in the vicious circle of binge eating to comfort eat.

When I was 30 I reached breaking point in a long-term relationship I was in; I had ballooned to more than 21 stone in weight. I was desperately unhappy and I knew I was the only person who could do anything about it. I also knew I had to break my ex-partners heart to make myself happy as he had become totally dependent on both me and cannabis and had begun to lead a life that was very dark. He was also cheating on me and had registered himself on some very disturbing websites looking for alternative encounters. He had also started to deal cannabis in order to fund his own habit and he would think nothing of spending £1000 a week on cannabis. It was during this time that I had a very early miscarriage; I didn't know I was pregnant and it came as a huge shock to me. I decided not to tell my partner about this as he was not emotionally stable enough to deal with such a situation. My periods also had an effect on this relationship as the constant bleeding affected the physical aspect of our relationship and it was apparently the reason that he 'had to look elsewhere for things'.

Over the years I had tried all sorts of medication and treatment to ease my periods and in the end just put up with what became the norm for me. I knew I had to lose weight for many reasons and I used the opportunity of a fresh start to do just that! I lost six stone, found a new confidence and zest for life yet there was still no let up with the bleeding. I was advised that the Mirena coil would be the cure I needed so I agreed to have one fitted; but I was not warned how painful it could be and I fainted very shortly after I had it fitted! I have a very high pain threshold and this pain was pretty intense, afterwards they told me it is more painful for women who have not had children. Nice warning!!

During this time I met and moved in with a new partner; he had two children and we had discussed having a baby together. This relationship was far from perfect and he had a very aggressive and angry side. There were signs that things were not right and very suddenly just before Christmas I found out that he had been seeing other men and sleeping with them in our bed whilst I was in work. I had no idea at all about this; I also had no idea that he was bisexual. That relationship ended very suddenly and without warning; I woke up one morning and within hours I found out I had been cheated on, that my partner was bisexual and I had been made homeless. This had a very bad affect on my confidence yet it was a huge relief to be out of such a volatile relationship. I was very grateful that my parents allowed me to move back in with them and in hindsight this really did happen for a reason.

I subsequently rebelled against being in such a bad relationship; I was angry at the world but even angrier with men. I became a little promiscuous which was very unlike me and I will admit to doing things I am ashamed of and deeply regret. I was getting some male attention and as my confidence was so low and I was very vulnerable, I gave in to my wilder side. I became intimate with a guy I had met on a free internet dating website; we had met for coffee a few times and decided to take things a little further. We booked into a hotel and I started unexpectedly flooding which was becoming the norm for me. The bleeding just would not stop and was very, very heavy; the poor man really freaked out and tried to call an ambulance for me! I reassured him that I would be okay and asked him to kindly take me home. It was very embarrassing and I never saw or heard from him again. I saw my GP the following morning and yet again was re-referred back to the gynaecologist.

I was starting to notice changes in my body and I developed a band of dark skin around my neck and on my chest; I became so self conscious about this that I scrubbed at it with a nail brush and tried my best to cover it with makeup, but I still could not cover it. I was getting to the point where I just could not cope with not only the pain of my periods but the way it was affecting my life. I was really enjoying a new found freedom; I had a good circle of friends and was really enjoying my life; I actually enjoyed being single. The only blight was my periods. There were times where all I could do was lie in bed with plastic bags and towels underneath me as every time I moved, I flooded. I was spending a small fortune on sanitary towels and always had a change of underwear with me.

I had a hysteroscopy in March 2010 and I was told that the results from a biopsy of my womb were nothing to worry about. My family saw how much I suffered and in July 2010 I made the heart-breaking decision that I would have a hysterectomy. Although my consultant was reluctant, he agreed to undertake the procedure as he understood that I had tried every treatment option and had also witnessed my suffering. I was 33 years old, I hadn't had children and I was single.

I had remained friends with my ex-partner who offered to try for a baby with me before I had the hysterectomy; I politely declined his offer for many, many reasons!

I wasn't given much time to prepare myself for the hysterectomy which I was very glad about, I spent the two weeks before like a zombie yet the morning of the procedure an unbelievable calm came over me. I very clearly recall my consultant asking me while I was waiting in theatre reception if I was 100% sure I wanted to go ahead with the procedure as it was a huge responsibility not only for him but for the hospital to take. I knew deep down that there was something seriously wrong with me, call it gut instinct or women's intuition, and I insisted that he went ahead with the procedure.

The hysterectomy did not go according to plan and I was in theatre and recovery for almost eight hours. I was discharged from hospital two days early on more than 30 tablets a day and had I also had to give myself injections each day. A few days after discharge my wound split and I got an infection; double antibiotics didn't clear up the infection and district nurses had to visit me daily for two weeks to dress my wound. I felt like I had left my dignity at the hospital door the day I had my hysterectomy.

I felt so ill after the hysterectomy and it came as a huge shock to me, I had not expected to feel half as bad as I did. They say pets can sense emotions, I had never got on very well with my mum's cat Cassius and we generally gave each other a very wide berth. I was so tired and fed up of being ill that one day when I was on my own I just sat at the table and sobbed, Cassius came and sat underneath me and rubbed her head against my leg and stayed there until I had stopped crying. I think we shared a moment that day.

I was told that I would be followed up three months after the hysterectomy; when I received a letter from the hospital four weeks later asking me to see my consultant the following day; I kind of guessed I would be receiving bad news. My parents took me to my appointment as I wasn't able to drive yet; my dad waited in the car; he still finds women's problems difficult to deal with. After a three hour wait I sat down with my gynaecology consultant at the end of his clinic, he put his hand on mine and told me I had endometrial cancer. Nothing can really prepare you to hear those dreaded words. I managed to hold myself together pretty well while I was in the consultation room; I don't remember an awful lot about what I was being told but I do remember the poor medical student sitting in the corner of the room looking very uncomfortable as my mum and I sat in stunned shock.

I came out of the consultation room and absolutely crumbled; my mum was heartbroken but was trying so hard to stay strong for me. We met my dad outside and I sobbed on him, we have never been a particularly demonstrative family yet he just held me and we all cried together. I cry every time I think of this as the memory is so vivid, I still can't walk past the bench outside the hospital without crying because of the memory.

I went back to the hospital a few days later to meet the oncology consultant and team and to find out my treatment options. As it was extremely rare for someone of my age to get womb cancer I was asked to take part in a number of genetics studies. I felt like I was pounced upon and asked to sign a mountain of forms giving my consent for tissue samples to be sent around the country. It also felt like gallons of blood were taken from me; the irony!

I consider myself very fortunate that I didn't have to have any further treatment; the hospital was fairly sure that the cancer had been contained. My fallopian tubes and one and a half ovaries were kept in situ and assurances were made to me that the cancer had not spread and was very unlikely to have spread. An agreement was made that I would have ultrasound scans and follow-up in oncology clinic every three months in order to monitor me.

I don't really feel that I fit in anywhere with my diagnosis; when I attend my oncology appointments I am the youngest person in the waiting room. I have attended a few support groups run by the hospital for women with gynaecological cancers but again I am the youngest person there, the average age is about 55 and the way womb cancer affects someone my age, and a woman who is post-menopause is pretty different. I feel like an outsider when I am at these groups. However I received a very encouraging letter recently informing that they are considering starting a support group for women under the age of 45. I am so excited at the prospect I have even volunteered to help run the support group!

All I have ever wanted is to have a child of my own and I can honestly say that making the decision to have the hysterectomy was the hardest thing I have ever had to do. I still beat myself up about this even two and a half years post-op. I haven't held a baby since I had my hysterectomy and friends and colleagues do treat me differently; I have found that people are afraid of upsetting me by telling me they are pregnant or even talking about babies. This makes me feel even worse and I often refer to myself as a freak because of it.

I have found that since I had cancer people treat me differently too, I don't feel like I am me anymore, I have almost lost my identity. Some people just didn't know how to talk to me and I lost some friends because of it. When I was diagnosed my ex-partner, who asked me to have a baby with him, decided to tell me that he loved me; we had been together for a year before we split and he had never even told me he liked me, never mind loved me. I think cancer affects others in a variety of ways. One friend took my diagnosis far harder than I did and used it as an opportunity to gain attention. I just wanted to carry on as I was before but it was very difficult to be allowed too.

Following my diagnosis my GP referred me to a holistic centre that I fondly refer to as the 'knitting nanas'. The support and treatment I received from them was amazing; I was given Indian head massages, acupuncture and had a few sessions of counselling. I was advised to start writing a journal which I have kept and when I read back some of the things that I have written when I was at my lowest, I don't recognise the person I am reading about. Something that really jumps out at me is 'if I took an overdose of antidepressants, would I die happy?' I feel so sad when I read that because I realise just how low I had become; I am a bright bubbly person and I try so hard not to let things get to me and just get on with my life as best I can.

I was battling so many of my own demons, yet I was carrying the guilt that I had chosen to have the hysterectomy, taken away my own fertility and that I had taken the privilege of grandchildren away from my parents. But I was also carrying the burden of having cancer and knowing I had something so evil growing inside of me. I was trying to stay so strong for my parents because they were absolutely devastated that their daughter had cancer; I felt so guilty that I was putting others through emotions I had no control over. I was frustrated that I wasn't able to look after myself physically and that I had become a burden to people. I had gone from being a fiercely independent person who worked full time and had a brilliant social life, to someone who could not even make a cup of tea. I suppose as a coping mechanism I blocked out a lot of my emotions in order to try and recover physically; I put my own emotions on the backburner but eventually they came to the surface.

It took about 18 months but I eventually had what I refer to as a meltdown, and it was quite an impressive one! I work in mental health for a consultant psychiatrist, I get on with her extremely well and she knew I was very low so suggested that I saw her colleague who was also an oncology psychiatrist. I was given an appointment to see her rather quickly and it was very refreshing to talk to someone who didn't know me and who I could be brutally honest with about my feelings. I was told it was entirely normal to feel the way I did and I was referred for CBT. In the beginning I found this extremely useful, but I felt I was being overwhelmed by appointments. I was being seen by geneticists, oncologists and therapists. I felt like I was being weighed down by cancer and I just wanted to escape it. It took a few months but I just made a pact with myself to just carry on with my life and accept everything that had been dealt to me.

There is nothing I can do to change what has happened so I just deal with it the best way I know how, with a sense of humour! I find that although I don't have periods anymore, my brain and my body are in battle with each other. I still get period pains and have mood swings, but knowing that there is a pattern to them makes it easier to deal with as I know I won't feel low forever.

There are days when out of the blue reality hits and I realise I will never have the little girl I have longed for and I will cry for the baby I will never hold. But I am also thankful that I am still alive.

Having cancer can be very difficult on a relationship. I briefly had a relationship with a guy who I met on a dating website a few months after the hysterectomy. It was hard physically and mentally; he hadn't seen the struggles I had been through or how difficult it had been for me and I will never forget him telling me that I just had to 'man up and get on with it'. That pretty much put the nail in that relationship coffin! I made a vow to myself after that that I would never ever meet anyone from a dating website ever again! I could write a whole new story about the scrapes I got myself into through internet dating!

I was on a very rare night out with my best friend; we had both had a bad week and decided that we needed to let our hair down! I never in a million years expected to meet anyone; I just wanted a carefree night out! We were in my favourite rock club and I saw a guy looking at me, and being the person I am, thought he was about to shout at me! But we got chatting and we have been together ever since! I decided that I needed to be totally honest with him about the cancer and hysterectomy; he took it really well and just accepts me the way I am. We are living together now and it appears that our paths have crossed many times through the years without us ever knowing each other as we have mutual friends! Fate is very strange indeed.

I count myself very fortunate that I didn't have to have radiotherapy or chemotherapy following the hysterectomy. I was assured that the cancer was very unlikely to have spread, however I will never ever feel that I am free of cancer.

Knowing that I had been walking around with a monster inside me without even knowing about it still scares me. So many people have told me how brave I am, how I am an inspiration and how strong I am; but I feel as though they are talking about someone else. I am nothing special, I was just dealt a tough blow and I chose to deal with it the only way I know how, head on.

I was at a concert recently and I as looked around me it occurred to me that we all have our own lives yet strangers don't know about the struggles we face. I was just a face in a sea of people, yet I feel cancer is my dirty secret.

Recovery Is The Secret To Success, Susan Carman

Back in February 2007 my uterus was removed (actually in my opinion it was only a vessel). I had reached the new 30 (50) and ever since I had my daughter back in 1976 I have had a prolapse. Together with ever decreasing oestrogen levels, years of top-level horse training and competing, large baby (forceps delivery) episiotomy and a 'new husband' on my 50th birthday everything went south; including my bladder!

I never made it to the loo in time, wore pads constantly and felt generally uncomfortable, taking to the bushes when exercising our beagles. A ring pessary alleviated the problem, but it made intercourse interesting to say the least! It is possible! However this is no laughing matter at my young age, after all I'm a fit bird.

So surgery was the answer, 'better out than in', I say.

After waiting six months as quoted (the length of time for this op on the waiting list) I went in for the op. First on the list, great, super service from the NHS staff; anaesthetic (like having too many gin & tonic's); best sleep I have ever had, woke up later, no pain at all. Discovered they had removed it vaginally as planned, and repaired the cystocele (collapse of front wall of vagina pushing bladder out of place), great!

Went in Friday, out Sunday morning, no pain. No blood. A drain was in and a catheter but you could not really tell. This was removed Saturday and I was delighted. The best op I have ever had. Now I have broken lots of bones in my time but this was no more than a tooth out girls. You have to be really positive about this it is a new lease of life! Even on my six week check-up, he didn't peek! No need, I gave the very handsome chap the thumbs up. If you have finished with the vessel it is the kindest cut of all for woman.

Okay, I am taking low dose HRT but this is fantastic. A vaginal op is the way to go! I now have a designer vagina and am back in the saddle! Within a week I was walking our pack – I believe walking to be the best therapy for life, after all you are a long time on your back!

So, a year passed and all was well – weight down although never fat, life continued and then out of the blue, something not quite right down below! I found emptying my bowel difficult and time consuming whereas prior I was always regular and no trouble. So off to the GP I went and guess what 'a rectocele' was diagnosed! What is it? It's a bulge of the back passage drops into your vagina like a bend so the waste has to enter the bend before exiting out through the rectum – causing constipation and sluggish motions! So like a cystocele it has to be stitched up and repaired (surgery).

This I underwent under general anaesthesia; again a six week recovery. At the post-op check it was thumbs up and job done (pardon the pun!). Now here we are in 2013 and guess what, I need more surgery! I have a grade three cystocele!

The front wall of the vagina has collapsed. Great! It's also causing incontinence again as it's difficult to control muscles therein. I can do pelvic floor exercises and have done so regularly, even before any ops. I believe that:

a) it is not always the best way forward to do a 'repair' at the same time as a vaginal hysterectomy; the two must be separate.

b) any stretching of the delicate tissues can compromise ability to go back to normality.

c) my lifestyle and recovery probably dictates the best practice as I have 11 beagles and life is full on.

I do believe you must take time out for at least six weeks. No lifting, pushing, pulling, hoovering, carrying, shopping bag carrying! I saw a consultant again and had a bladder scan – revealing I could not empty totally so had the urethra stretched (not painful). This helped somewhat and shows we need oestrogen for collagen and elasticity.

Unfortunately since I had this done months ago, I have seen the consultant privately who performed the successful rectocele and I am on his NHS list for the cystocele repair although, if the wait is too lengthy, I will pay privately and could have the op as early as next week!

So in conclusion, things can go awry but this is my individual story and you must stay positive as we are all different. Your hysterectomy is personal to you and if I had one piece of advice it is keep calm, feet up, recovery is the secret to success!

A Very Happy Hysterectomy, Fe Cleeson

Hi Ladies (and gentlemen) I had a TAH and BSO on 3rd December 2012. As with many of us my route to a hysterectomy was long, painful and at times frustrating. I had been suffering with heavy periods for some years and had tried, unsuccessfully, to get some sort of relief with my symptoms.

Following an ultrasound scan, I was diagnosed with a large ovarian cyst. I was then referred to a consultant gynaecologist, who was very reluctant to perform a hysterectomy. After several appointments with my GP and re-referral's to the hospital, I asked to be referred to another consultant.

I was admitted to hospital on 3rd December for the operation. I have nothing but praise for the treatment I received. Everyone was fabulous. My new consultant was so kind, gentle and professional. I was given all the information I needed to make an informed choice and at this time we both agreed a hysterectomy was the best decision for me. I have a very low pain threshold and can't take morphine so a PCA pump was a non starter! Plus I am the world's biggest coward when it comes to pain! It did hurt when I first came round but after that the rest of the day and night seemed to pass in a blur.

By Tuesday I was able to eat and drink, so I could take Ibuprofen again, which was the best pain killer for me. By Wednesday I was up and about – sore but nowhere near as painful as I thought it would be. Everything went very smoothly with no complications.

I came home on the Friday. Within a week I was out and about – a short walk to the local shop was exhausting but manageable. I was amazed at how much I could do so soon after. I was sensible and have a very caring partner who nagged me constantly about doing too much! I even managed to cook Christmas dinner!

Four months on and I am back at work, still tired but am so happy with the results of my surgery. I am pain free, period free and feel like I can actually start to live again after years of debilitating pain and bleeding.

I am having a few problems with the menopause – it hit me like a brick on the 1st January, with all the usual symptoms – severe night sweats, mood swings, depression, joint pains. Although it is difficult, I try to remind myself that I am very lucky to have had such a great experience with my surgery.

If you are reading this and thinking something along the lines of 'who does she think she is, Superwoman?' Please let me explain that I was 48 when I had my operation. I have type-two diabetes, arthritis, hypothyroidism and depression. I am also obese – one reason why my first consultant didn't want to perform a hysterectomy. I had lost some weight, having being diagnosed with diabetes, but will always struggle with food.

What I wanted to say here was that I have read some very sad stories and I know how lucky I am to have been treated so well both in hospital and at home.

So what have I found out about all this? Ladies, we are all different, unique individuals. Although we may be having the same or similar types of surgery, be kind to yourselves. Your body and your mind will heal in their own way and at their own pace. There is no right or wrong way to feel or to recover – just take time to find your own way through it. And don't be hard on yourself – take your time to find what works for you. And if you're not happy with the way you're treated, speak up. You wouldn't take your car to a garage where you didn't trust the mechanic, so why put your body in the hands of someone you aren't comfortable with?

Thank you so much for the '101 Handy Hints for a Happy Hysterectomy' book – it really did help; as did the fabulous, if less than glamorous support pants. The nurses loved the book. And I still wear the support pants when I go for a long walk or a trip to the gym – my scar is still a little sore at times. Plus they keep the cold out –

very important during the long Cumbrian winter!! So, that's why I have called my story 'A Very Happy Hysterectomy' and I hope yours will be too.

Two and Half Years Post-Op Total Abdominal Hysterectomy, Liz

Well ladies what can I say? I used the website a lot initially after my op and was always optimistic I would be okay.

How wrong I was.

I am not able to take HRT (history of breast cancer in family, and abnormal cells found earlier this year – so it`s definitely a no-no.

I am still experiencing these symptoms: sweats (GP giving acupuncture which I do think has helped), sleep problems, irritability and low mood (especially with partner), no libido, vaginal dryness, pain in joints (ankles/elbows and fingers – especially in the morning), weight gain (2 stone – or 28lbs). I have had several falls in the past two and half years so I have asked for a bone density scan to make sure I don`t need supplements for bones as well.

I am taking linseed/flaxseed oil and very recently started vitamin B6 (before succumbing to anti-depressants)!

In the past two and half years years I have experienced the following which I think have not helped my symptoms:

June 2010 – total abdominal hysterectomy

July 2010 – mother given terminal prognosis

September 2010 – mother died

September 2010 – supporting father

October 2010 – November 2010 – receiving counselling

December 2011 – father had heart attack

March 2012 – father seriously ill.

May 2012 – father discharged from hospital

May 2012 – July 2012 – supporting father to better health

July 2012 – Mammogram

August 2012 – recalled for mammogram and biopsy

September 2012 – operation to remove abnormal breast cells

September 2012 – low mood, irritability and depression?

November 2012 – new job (secondment until March 2013)

December 2012 – daughter lost pregnancy

For those ladies reading this before your op my advice is to get as much information as possible and don't be afraid to ask your doctor or consultant. I didn`t and wished I had, so I had an informed choice. I will always regret my hysterectomy because I wasn`t convinced I needed it in the first place.

The 'Alien' Is Removed, Sally

In June 2011 my GP felt a large mass in my abdomen so I was referred to a gynaecologist. On an ultrasound one of my ovaries couldn't be seen so I had an MRI to check it wasn't ovarian cancer and luckily it wasn't; I had a large subserosal fibroid and two tiny ones. The consultant explained about hysterectomy, myomectomy and leaving the fibroid in situ. I later asked about embolisation. Initially I opted for a hysterectomy and he said I could decide on the day of my op whether or not to keep my ovaries. I said I'd have my cervix removed as I'd had abnormal smears in 2009, although not serious ones.

I then looked on-line in an attempt to make an informed decision. Although the large fibroid measured 16cm x 11cm x 8cm I had very few symptoms, mainly bloating, no pain or heavy bleeding. My op was scheduled for November 11th but I still had many questions. I'd read that a hysterectomy should be the last resort. I was very confused. If I had bad symptoms the decision would have been easier. There were so many unknowns and a lot to consider. One thing I did decide early on was to keep my ovaries because I wanted the testosterone after menopause. My surgeon decided to cancel/postpone the surgery hours before my pre-op as he could tell

I was unsure of my decision. At no point did he suggest what I should do. It was up to me to decide with my layman's knowledge!

Early 2012 I wanted a myomectomy, a much bloodier operation but I didn't want a blood transfusion. I worried that the two small fibroids might grow if I went on to HRT to reduce the hot flushes that were disturbing my sleep (I am now using natural progesterone cream for hot flushes but that too can apparently make large fibroids grow!).

In April I saw a lady registrar who told me that most women, even with a large fibroid, left it in situ if they weren't getting problems. I discussed with her concerns about sexual function. She told me there are nerves in your cervix that can affect your orgasm and I'd also read this online. She suggested that, should I need surgery in future, to have a sub-total hysterectomy. Great! Decision made to leave the 'alien' in!

Symptoms and hormone tests in January showed I was peri-menopausal so it was unlikely to grow unless I took HRT! Three weeks later I looked pregnant (not good at 49) and I had my first period for five months. A new test showed my hormone levels were in the normal range. I had another ultrasound which suggested the fibroid had grown so I opted for a sub-total hysterectomy.

I've not had children but that wasn't the real concern. I struggled with so much contradictory information and the fact that we are all different. There were so many uncertainties. I was scared about weight gain post-op and being unable to lose it as many women seem to experience this. I've mainly been slim which is why looking bloated was a problem for me. I was also worried about orgasms being affected. Right up to the day of the op I was considering cancelling. What got me there in the end was that I might still be wondering what to do for years to come and I needed closure. My inability to make a decision was causing me a lot of anxiety despite asking friends and family to help me decide. Maybe I was too informed!

I joined a gym in June to get fitter and I lost half a stone. I had the op early October and it went well. I hardly used the PCA; I didn't get an infection and kept wind at bay by drinking peppermint tea! One week post-op I went into town for an hour.

My energy levels were amazingly good. Five months post-op my lower abdomen is still numb and sometimes feels uncomfortable. My scar is neat and tidy. I haven't gained weight. Orgasms are fine but I don't know if that would have been the case if I'd not kept my cervix. Pre-op I saw several doctors hoping to make what has been one of the hardest decisions of my life.

The fibroid hadn't grown but at least it's gone now. I asked for a photo of my fibroid so if I had any problems post-op and wondered why I'd had the operation with so few symptoms, I could look at it and tell myself that's why!

Why Me! Sharon Loft

My story starts in 2003; I was trying for a baby and suddenly started to get heavy periods. Why Me!

Despite my self pity, I am happy to say in 2005 my son was born and when my period returned they were normal. Over the next few years I started to bleed extremely heavily again and my periods became irregular so I finally went to my Dr's when I couldn't cope anymore. This was February 2012. After a referral to a consultant, and a laparoscopic investigation I was advised I needed a total hysterectomy. Why Me! Luckily I found the Hysterectomy Association and found it wasn't just happening to me.

In June 2012 I was admitted to hospital to have my op by keyhole surgery. I went down to the theatre at 8.30am expecting to be back in my room by 11am however, I woke up in the recovery room at 5.30pm being told I was being transferred to another hospital's high dependency unit as I had been on the operation table so long and I had also lost a lot of blood. When I finally came around fully, I found out that during the operation my bladder had been stuck to the bits being extracted. Why Me! Apparently, this is quite common in women whom have had a caesarean section.

The surgeon had to revert to open surgery and the urologist had to try to fix my bladder. I had two catheters inserted to ensure that my bladder was kept completely empty and I had to have a blood transfusion. After two nights I was transferred back to my original hospital where I stayed for another five days. I was finally discharged, with the two catheters and told my bladder should heal in three weeks. I was glad when the three weeks was over as life with catheters is not nice, the urethra one was so uncomfortable!!

D Day came and I went to the hospital for my bladder scan, looking forward to getting rid of the catheters only to be told my bladder still had a hole in it! Bladders apparently are very good a self-healing but mine seemed to be taking its time. Why Me!

I was sent away for another four weeks of sheer hell with the catheters, only to find out I still had a hole! I was then booked in for another op to re-fix the hole in my bladder, this time it was done by keyhole surgery. I was sent home for another four weeks and yes you've guessed right, it was still not fixed!!

Finally, at the end of November I went for my last scan before the consultant decided what action to take next as my bladder didn't appear to want to heal itself. This time the radiologist came out smiling... the hole had self healed. Despite reserved worries about how my bladder would work after being 'flat' for five months, boy did it feel good when the catheters came out.

After a long five months of mixed emotions; feeling sorry for myself asking 'Why me' I can almost put this episode of my life behind me. My bladder is almost back to normal, I have had no complications from the hysterectomy and the HRT injection is working a treat. My belly mind you is like a patch work quilt, with a new patch being added every six months for the HRT injection but I have stopped feeling sorry for myself and asking 'Why Me!'

Celebrating With A Meal And Present, Diane

It's hard to believe but I have just celebrated my second anniversary of my operation. Yep, CELEBRATED, as I have been healthy and back to 'babe' as my husband would say.

We even celebrate with a meal and I get a prezzie as well! Oh God how mad does that sound but after 12 years of hell and a very long emotional road, I am now getting on with life without being ruled by pain and heavy bleeding.

My story starts in my mid-30s when it became apparent something was wrong, and as we had been unable to have children I was now dealing with another problem, and so the trips to the doctors started.

Ten years later, living on the acid pills as I called them and my best friends the hormone pills, the expense of buying towels (my Boots Advantage Card Points soared!), I finally made the point to my GP that I couldn't go on in this state.

So two gynaecologists later (we moved house in between) lots of pills, an infection and a blood transfusion later I went to see my consultant again knowing there would only be one option.

That option I knew would be a hysterectomy; my womb was so stretched, my consultant suggested a fibroid tumour but he couldn't be sure. As I have private medical insurance it was time to use it so I rang to book my operation. How weird was that? It was like booking concert tickets which would have been preferable. My date was set six weeks away in June. My choice as I had so much work on, which I put before my health! I had to double up on all my pills. I was all set; then my emotional roller-coaster started and boy did it. I seemed to be on a treadmill of not 'being a woman anymore', how would it affect my marriage (Andy was fantastic), the impossibility of having children would turn over in my head. I would be hormonal all the time. I would cry alone – did I really need this operation?

Being a retail manager my job keeps me very busy but I felt so alone. My friends and family were great but they only saw a poorly girl. I couldn't talk to anyone although I read lots about the operation and from the Hysterectomy website – the chat rooms were so helpful. I began to think it was me. The strange thing during all this was that I had no symptoms and felt well, so well in fact I cancelled my operation! I would be fine, I didn't need this.

Two weeks later I haemorrhaged badly at work. My blood levels dropped so much that I needed a blood transfusion; I could barely walk or function. It was then that I had a talk with my excellent GP, rebooked my operation and this time I was all set. No going back now!

The day dawns and we drive through a bad thunderstorm to the hospital. Was this an omen? My operation took longer than expected, as I was due to have key-hole surgery which couldn't be done due to the size of my womb, so my consultant had to make the decision to do it openly, which he told me when I woke up, not that I really cared. I even had some photos of my womb, one for the album!

I recovered really well and enjoyed my time off. I work full time so the break and some good weather really helped. But I never forget my emotional road and even now it does sometimes drop back in to see me.

I am lucky and so well, I feel a 1000 times better so as hard as it all was, you can come out of this a new woman.

Fibroids And Polycystic Ovaries, Karen

After suffering for many years from fibroids and polycystic ovary syndrome my gynaecologist finally decided it was time to go for the hysterectomy option. I had already gone down the path of medication and microwave ablation twice and whilst it offered short term relief it wasn't long before the symptoms reared their ugly heads again; the worst being the constant and heavy bleeding and the pain.

Being only 42 at the time and recently divorced it was quite a blow, I was worried about the obvious effects of early menopause, would I still feel like a woman, would I still be able to have a fulfilling sex life, orgasm etc.?

Everything was prepared in advance, hormone replacement discussed, and assurances given that my life should be much improved by the operation. My gynae opted for a full hysterectomy using the laparoscopic technique with epidural pain relief and I have to say that I was astounded by how well I felt when I came round. I was only in hospital for three days and although I felt tired and uncomfortable the pain was minor and I made a full a speedy recovery going back to work after eight weeks.

The operation made a huge difference to my life, nearly a year on I feel invigorated and not in the least bit unsexy or un-woman like. I have a fantastic sex life with a good and understanding man who understood my initial fear and was patient and considerate. And the other upside was that the hormone replacement seemed to kick my body back into life (after years of suffering from polycystic ovaries) and I managed to shed a couple of stones without even really trying.

People even tell me that I look somehow younger; I believe that this is because for the first time in several years I'm no longer in pain or drained of energy from the heavy periods. I feel and look better now than I have for years and the kids (I have four) say how great it is to have their happy go lucky mum back at long last.

Having a hysterectomy was for me the best decision and I hope my story gives hope and inspiration to other women on the brink of making the same decision.

Hysterectomy And Endocrine Problems, Mary

Although there were a few setbacks on the way to surgery, my surgery and initial recovery went far better than expected. Because of various existing health conditions my hysterectomy and unrelated bowel reconstruction were done under a single anaesthetic with two teams of surgeons at a specialist centre some distance (90 miles along country roads) from my home. I was discharged exactly a week after my surgery.

Three days after I got home my blood pressure started to drop and soon reached a dangerously low level. I'd had endocrine problems in the past so I knew what was happening, and what needed to be done. The emergency doctor came straight to the house and after a brief examination; he took baseline bloods and gave me an injection (a massive dose of drugs that acts as a cushion until more appropriate treatment can be started) then arranged admission to my local (very small) general hospital. I had suggested a larger hospital but he ruled I was not well enough to travel so far in safety. No ambulance was available so I went by car.

On arrival at the local hospital I was admitted to a general ward, which was both busy and quite dirty. I complained the toilet was not clean and was handed a cloth with which to clean it! This was just a few days after surgery and I had a barely healed wound.

I handed over the findings of the emergency doctor and the endocrinal crisis pack that I carry. My blood pressure was taken –

very low. This was the only time my blood pressure was taken during my time in this hospital. I was not allowed food (and more important drinks) until I had seen the doctor.

After four hours I saw a staff doctor. He phoned a larger hospital for advice and told me they would need to do x, y and z. I said I knew that already as it was an immediate requirement as stated in my emergency pack – he had not been given this and my situation was obviously well out of his depth. I asked for fluids and he looked shocked; with my endocrine crisis I should have been given lots of fluids to keep me hydrated and I was now at risk of kidney damage. He took another blood sample and took that sample and the ones taken by the emergency doctor to the lab.

Nothing else happened for a further two hours when I buzzed for a nurse and asked what was happening. 'Oh, you have been discharged. I'll find your letter.' So during my six hours in hospital I had scrubbed a toilet, had my blood pressure taken once, had a single blood sample taken and had risked kidney damage. I went home.

The next day my GP phoned very early – probably as soon as he got in. He said I was to come down to the surgery immediately, dressed or not, and we had to park in the space marked reserved for emergencies. My dear husband was to use a wheelchair to bring me in. I wasn't feeling too well at all and my GP gave me another massive dose of support drugs by injection. He phoned the local hospital and then the larger hospital. It was decided that I would continue with daily jabs until a specialist could see me. Later that day I had abdominal pain and took up residence in the loo. The trips for the daily jabs became a nightmare as the abdominal pain got worse and in desperation my GP and my husband decided to phone the unit where my surgery had been done. I was re-admitted. The drugs I was being given had to be discontinued as they were affecting my blood chemistry and my blood pressure fell again. I was confined to a bed with cot sides.

Samples showed I had picked up Norovirus and a call to the local hospital confirmed they had an outbreak in the ward both before and after I had been there. Great! After a lot of blood and other samples had been taken I was asked if I wanted to stay in or go home. I elected to go home – a big error on my part.

The following day I was still in pain. I took the maximum dose of pain killers, used heat pads, and a TENS machine. I tried to sleep. By the next morning I was suffering the most pain I had ever experienced. My husband rang the specialist unit and they said to come right in. I was rushed into the gynae A&E and then off for scans. I am not sure how many people can get into a standard ultrasound booth but we were certainly playing sardines as one person after another was called to have a look at the screen. They found a partially blocked kidney, an internal bleed and a massive collection. My temperature was rising and it was decided that the CT scan would have to be done immediately.

During my scans the paperwork had been done for me to be re-admitted to the ward. I no longer had a choice as by this time as my temperature was dangerously high and I was starting to fit and hallucinate.

An emergency call went out for a specialist radiologist to insert a drain into the collection. This was successful and the collection was found to contain about a pint of grot. The drain was left in place. I had drips inserted in just about anywhere you could imagine (and a few places you can't!) but I only have the haziest memories of this time. I was told later that things were very much in the balance and could have gone either way. Luckily I pulled through and was discharged after another week.

I still had both the endocrine problem and a blood chemistry problem but they could be held in check with bed rest until I saw a local endocrinologist and haematologist. I was only to be allowed out of bed to visit the loo until I had been seen.

When I got home I found I had missed the endocrinologist's outpatient appointment at the local hospital – it had been scheduled for whilst I was in the specialist unit. My DH phoned to explain but was told that as I had missed the appointment I would be put on the bottom of the waiting list. So two months after my hysterectomy I am still waiting for my endocrinology and haematology appointments. I can and do sit up in bed although it makes me very light headed. When I stand my blood pressure falls so much I faint. I need a wheelchair to get to the loo and back.

Am I pleased with the hysterectomy and glad I had it done? I think the surgeons did a brilliant job and regard the scar is a badge of honour. I have made a formal complaint about my local hospital and have had the standard letter back. I will be taking things further – to the SPSO (Scottish Public Services Ombudsman) if necessary. The tests I have had done indicate big problems within my endocrine system and my own knowledge tells me this will not wait for months to be sorted out

It is now about 10 months since my hysterectomy. I have been in and out of hospital during that time because of complications from both the surgery and the effect the surgery had on my existing health problems. I am waiting to be well enough to undergo further surgery and hope that may happen later this year (2013). I have already been told that this next lot of surgery will have a drastic affect on my life-style but if I don't have the surgery my health will deteriorate further. All I have read in medical texts back up the rather poor prognosis.

My feelings about the hysterectomy are very mixed. At the time a hysterectomy appeared to be the best choice for me but looking back I wish I had gone on asking about how my existing health conditions would affect the surgery and recovery, and how the surgery and recovery would affect my existing health problems. When I did ask the questions they were either avoided or I was told I was worrying unnecessarily. It is easy to look back and say 'I should have...' or 'I wish I had...' but that does not help the present situation and what I have is what I have to live with. I have a choice – to be a victim, sit and sob or to face the future with courage and determination. I choose the latter.

Many people have been very kind and people I hardly knew have helped my family and me through this difficult time whilst some of those I thought were good friends didn't even phone to find out how things had gone.

I no longer work and it is possible that I will not be employed again.

Life is Good, Pam

In 2006, I broke my ankle and was confined to the sofa for six weeks with my leg up and no exercise. Afterwards, I started to go to the gym as soon as possible to lose some of the weight I had put on. After a few weeks I thought I had pulled a muscle in my stomach and reluctantly went to the GP when it was not getting better of its own accord.

Within days I had an ultrasound scan, a CT scan and an appointment with a consultant. I now realised it was much more serious than a pulled muscle. In fact, by the next week I was in hospital having a 28lb ovarian tumour removed; I'd had no idea and no other symptoms.

I agreed to have a full hysterectomy as well and in fact the tumour turned out to be a borderline cancer so it was a very good decision for me. The first few days after the surgery went by in a bit of a blur, it was certainly a most uncomfortable and less than dignified experience, but made bearable by my fabulous consultant and the nursing staff. 12 weeks recovery and time off work was also much needed. I get angry when I read anything about less time being acceptable.

I had never really thought or read much about hysterectomy, assuming that at the age of 47 it was still something that happened to older people and not my concern. My physical recovery was at the rate to be expected and I had no specific problems. On the mental side, I did wonder how I would be affected but since my natural attitude is very practical and I 'just get on with it', I can honestly say that I have had very few negative thoughts.

I am all but past child bearing age, I don't miss my periods one bit and I was delighted to have lost so much weight so quickly and be able to treat myself to lots of new clothes. Of course, with a 12 inch vertical scar now, bikinis are out, but since I haven't worn one for 30 years, I'll live with that.

On a serious note though, don't imagine from this that my brush with cancer has not affected me. Who knows what the future could bring but I am just grateful to be able to carry on with my life and

I'm keen to support any activity to promote better awareness of ovarian cancer.

Since 2007 I had successful check-ups with my consultant every six months for five years and was given the final all clear a couple of years back. I have never looked back and have not had a single sick day off work since. Life is good.

A Grandmother's Tale: One Year On! Mary

I am 55 yrs. old and had a TAH with removal of ovaries and cervix a year ago. I had been experiencing 10 years of difficult pre menopause symptoms and had grown several very large fibroids so I looked six months pregnant (not fun in my 50's and already a grandmother!), and had experienced severe bleeding and increasing pain for a long time, which restricted my life intensely and caused me many embarrassing and difficult times despite medication. I feel I should have had the op at least two years before, but good old NHS insisted I jump through their hoops of various treatments first, to justify the cost of hysterectomy...

My surgical experience was traumatic, good old NHS again! But to put that aside it's not been an easy year. I don't bleed any more, I don't have pain, but until very recently my energy levels have been poor, my mood fluctuating low to good, and my sex life (yes – I do have one! even being a Nana!) very different as much of the passion is gone for me, though I want to stress that I still enjoy it for it's loving intimacy and the pleasure my partner feels. Following surgical menopause I take huge doses of HRT which reduces symptoms most of the time... I still have very poor sensation around the scar and have learned to accept my new figure with flabby pot belly below the scar (still tons better than looking six months pregnant at my age!).

I stayed in a Travelodge last night, having booked a standard room at the last minute, only to find I was given a room with disabled facilities. Went into the bathroom and, whoosh! was emotionally taken straight back the hospital ward by the wet room floor, bars, and raised toilet seat.

It made me think – was it worth it all, because I still have symptoms despite the HRT. My body is scarred and altered, my sex life is quieter.

I have to say 'yes', but with qualifications. I am saddened by the loss of libido, saddened that I experienced an artificial menopause despite being 54! That my otherwise healthy body was subject to the surgical knife and bears the scars. I have my life back, I can go to work, go out to a restaurant, to the theatre etc. not stressed I may bleed uncontrollably any minute; I can go on a plane! I have significantly reduced pain. I can go anywhere with a small hand bag rather than a holdall with changes of clothes. I can walk for miles without puffing and panting! I don't need to plan for a loo stop every 30 minutes.

My life is altered and it is no fairy tale ending. But I would say, if you have the money go for it when the time is right for you, not waiting for when the NHS will grudgingly cough up. Do your research, challenge your surgeon to justify whether you should have cervix, ovaries removed, ask questions and don't be pushed into surgery until you are sure.

Then move on! Life is precious and there is a better life to be lived after hysterectomy! I look forward to my second anniversary – in the hope I won't even notice its passing and I wish the same for you.

The Uninsured, Tracy

Last year I was diagnosed with a fibroid, as this has probably been there for at least a couple of years I thought nothing of it in relation to travelling. In March I asked for a referral to a gynaecologist because of pain. In May I had a laparoscopy, which confirmed this fibroid and many other small ones.

Our yearly travel insurance policy has come up for renewal, during the renewal there were medical questions asked. The last one being had I been referred to or seen a consultant (or similar), to which I answered yes. I gave the information that they asked for, that I had a hysterectomy planned, why – for fibroids, heavy bleeding and constant pain.

I had contacted the insurance company a month ago to ask what happens, and was told to phone after the hysterectomy as cover could not be added until after the operation. I was advised that there would be an additional premium to cover the fibroids, without this I could not add the cover after the hysterectomy. When I queried this I was advised that things had changed late last year. This could have been missed as I had an ultrasound via my GP to diagnose the fibroid initially, and this would not have been covered in the questions the insurance company ask, and if I had not had a referral in progress it may have been missed and I would not have been covered.

In summary I would advise anyone who is diagnosed with a fibroid to check their travel insurance, and advise them accordingly otherwise if they have any treatment or complications in any way connected to gynae issues which leaves them unable to undertake a planned holiday, they may find themselves uninsured.

Finally Well After A Full Abdominal At 31, Nina

Like many girls, I started my periods at 11, but quickly realised that mine where different to others. The pain and blood loss were much higher than I could really cope with and still function. There is a history down my mothers and grandmothers side that this is how it has always been for 'us girls', so I tried to put up as best I could. By 15 I needed something to help and went to my doctor, he prescribed the pill for me, but my mother didn't want me to take it. It wasn't till much later she and I would understand why.

From 17 to 26 I became a testing ground for all doctors and sexual health doctors trying to control my periods and moods with the latest and the newest hormonal treatments. Over the years my mental and physical health deteriorated so much, I wanted nothing more than to end my life. My body had become so sensitive to anything that it came into contact with: foods, drinks, drugs. I had gained about four stone in fluid retention and bleed on average for 22 days out of 28. Because I bleed so much, my iron and potassium levels became dangerously low.

I come from a long line of women that don't give in though. Throughout this I never gave up work, relationships or training. Looking back, it nearly killed me, but did keep me sane also!

I knew in my heart at 18 that I wasn't going to have children, my body had told me this and so by 26, extremely ill and struggling with life begged doctors to take my womb away. They wouldn't, not until I was at least 30. Saying that I would change my mind about children and that if I did have one, it would probably get a lot better. This is what they told my grandma and mother, and it didn't work out well for them! So I thought hard and concluded that even if we (yes I had a long suffering partner, who is now my husband help me through all of this) did want children, I was far too ill to raise them, what were these doctors thinking?

Then the real dark years came, time of work with anxiety and depression. I was sleeping night after night on the bathroom floor unable to carry my own weight back to bed as it reacts to the day's assault of food and blood loss. I continued to try and seek medical help, but all they see is a jabbering wreck and put it all down to mental health issues. I wonder where the strong minded, high functioning, well educated person had gone, swallowed up completely by this body that could no longer function for more than a few days a month.

Finally I found a female GP who saw more than just the tears and 'period problems' and saw that there were real issues. She tried of course a few things, but quickly passed me on to a female gynae surgeon. At last I thought, but then the fear, how was I going to talk to her, I couldn't talk to anyone any more without being reduced to a jibbering snotty mess. So I wrote what I wanted to say, and for the first time in 10 years I felt like myself. I introduced myself and described how life had been. I added an insert from my then husband about his not wanting children and that we were very happy together, especially if I could gain my health back.

She read the letter in full before saying very much, looked at me with tears running down my face and asked how soon I would like the hysterectomy. Relief to finally be heard and taken seriously, I wasn't mad and unstable and secretly just depressed because I don't have children. So happy with this news I told a few friends, their shock horrified me. I then realised how well I had hid my ill health, and culturally women of breeding age fear and distrust those that say they do not want children of their own. So yet again I faced this without much support.

The hospital staff soon registered I was not a usual hysterectomy patient, as I was pumped with adrenaline and excitement. So much so they gave me sleeping tablets before my anaesthetic, which didn't work! I was in hospital for two nights, the staff were amazing and they soon worked out my pain thresholds, as I managed the post-op pain myself, never asking for pain killers, until it was suggested as my husband was about to visit and they thought it would be more comforting for him to see me in less distress. I have had other surgery and it was no more discomforting than that, not scary and from the minute I opened my eyes on the ward, I knew I would start feeling better again, not post surgical, but as a whole.

I didn't completely do as I was told when I got home, but you generally only make the mistake once and then you take it steadier. Feeling fit again and post surgical, knowing I needed to strengthen my stomach muscle, once I got the all clear I had healed, I swam daily to get my strength back. It felt great and didn't put the pressure on the stomach muscles that had been cut, so allowed them to heal and strengthen at the same time.

I returned to a very physical and demanding job after 12 weeks absence a new woman. Six months after my op I had glandular fever, I didn't know this until I dropped back into my doctors for blood test results, checking that my iron and potassium levels were now where they should be. She asked if I had been feeling unwell at all, I said a bit rough, sore throat but just put it down as a cold, she laughed and said how ill we're you before your op to say think that glandular fever is a slight cold.

And here I am five years on. The weight gain has all but gone and my mental health has been stable ever since. All of my allergies/sensitivities have gone and I have managed to put myself back on the career path I wanted, retraining and working hard. I do not ever regret my decision and know I never will, as I have my life back, my body back, my mind back and no child could have given me that.

Getting My Life Back After A Subtotal Hysterectomy, Paula Kirby

I had a subtotal hysterectomy on 29th December 2011 and now have my life back. I have suffered with very heavy periods all my life but especially since I had my children. My doctor was not very helpful and was quite rude about it saying it happens to all women and there was nothing that could be done.

Last October I had to have a health check because I reached 45 years of age and was told to lose weight. I should go swimming as that was the easiest way to lose it. After explaining to the nurse that I hadn't been swimming since my last son was born over 18 years ago because of the problems that I had she was rather angry that I had done nothing about it.

She made me go see the new female doctor who arranged everything and now I have my life back and can do anything without worrying about periods and leakage.

I Never Knew How Sick I Really Was, Sandi

Wow, I didn't realise how sick I was until I was six months post-op. I feel great since my hysterectomy. Oh it was a scary road, but well worth the travel. I am 47, excuse me 48 years old and have had painful periods since day one! 'Oh take the birth control pill', 'oh lose weight', 'oh no, take out my uterus, ovaries and tubes'!

I have more energy and life just in the six months since my surgery. Yes, it was painful and took a lot out of me, but now I have so much more. No more constant pain, worry about bleeding, cramps, and clots, or cancer! The doctor didn't even know how messed up my organs were until she went in to take them out!

I would still be in pain, oh, I don't want to think of where I would be now if I hadn't had it done. I did have to try a few different hormone replacement therapies and I didn't want to try any at first. But now I get a shot every four weeks and I feel great, great I tell you!

I will shout from the rooftops to have a hysterectomy to any one, and everyone I know who has had one done feels great and so full of life! I think it could be a requirement as soon as you hit a certain age, out they all go! I have had menstrual problems for over half of my life, wow, most of my life and I am living the rest of my life with a smile on my face! Thank you!

Goodbye My Lover! Ruiz Megan

I always had pain with my periods. I started mine when I was 10. I had painful sex. I put up with it, I even had problems having my children, but at the age of 34 I began having a swollen stomach, iron deficient and shortness of breath.

I saw a doctor recommend by my obstetrician and he said 'It's endometriosis and you have three kids – do you want more?' I didn't, I was tired of hurting and he said 'Okay, just take out the uterus, one ovary and the cervix all will be well and the best is the endometriosis will go away!'

I had my surgery and four days later I began to have severe back pain cough and sneezing, and I would leak urine! He sent me back to work two weeks later and all of my stuff dropped: bladder, bowels and vaginal cuff – it was a prolapse! He checked me at six weeks and said all is okay!

I told him my husband didn't want sex anymore and he said well you don't have sex with the uterus! I told him I had no feeling and he said it was in my head!

My job fired me and my husband wouldn't speak to me; he acted like I didn't deserve to breathe! So in 2008 I had reconstructive surgery and my doctor told me never to lift anything over three pounds or stand longer than one hour!

I haven't worked in so long and thank God for my son who took care of me, who gave me my meds and encouraged me to stay strong. There are not many 16 year old boys sleep on the floor by their mother's bed and run to get water or whatever I needed!

I have a grandson now he is 14 months old and it hurts so bad that I can't pick him up, hold him, take him to the park! I lost a lot. I loved my husband so much but he just turned his back on me and left me, just like that!

Today I'm 41 years old and I suffer in so many ways I cry a lot, I'm so mad that endometriosis does not ever go away but the doctor told me it would, he said it will all be done – no more! Every day I deal with this fear that if my bladder, bowels and vaginal cuff come down what do I do?

I have no money, I lost my home, my job, my husband and you know this nurse said 'well we can always just sew you up just like we do the old ladies'!

I'm not old, I'm not a freak! I want so desperately to not have had this surgery. I have thyroid disease and now my skin is wrinkled and my breasts just went south! My big butt is a flat butt with no hormones. I can't take it; I have chest pain and red spots on my legs! All this for what? I lost a lot!

I Didn't Have Time, Janet

My husband had been very ill for along time, and sadly died in 2010. I think my problems started around 2008 or before. I was looking after him, and he needed help to get around. When we went out at the beginning he used a small portable electric scooter. I was lifting it in and out of the car all the time, and they are not exactly light.

I have been a nurse all my life, and I have moved heavy patients and so on, so I didn't even think about the weight but it obviously didn't help. I was getting older and as a result of all the lifting I kind of realised that things were getting uncomfortable, but didn't do anything about it. I just put everything off as I didn't have time.

When my husband died I finally went to see about my problem. After various tests and appointments they decided on a hysterectomy. The website was excellent, it felt like a friend. I would tell other women not to wait like I did.

I had a vaginal hysterectomy and afterwards wondered why I had been so apprehensive as I have never looked back.

Severe Headache, Sharon Morris

I had a total hysterectomy on 7th December 2012 and everything went well. I was discharged on 10th December but on 16th December I was shopping in Tesco when I was suddenly struck with a blinding headache. It started on my left side and within minutes it had travelled across my whole forehead. I was sick, the pain was unbearable; I had never experienced anything like it.

I took two paracetamol and went to bed in a dark room to sleep it off but after two hours the pain was still ferocious. I was crying and being sick. My husband telephoned the hospital and they admitted me. I had to have an injection to rid me of the pain.

I was in hospital for a further two days still suffering the headache and my only relief was to lie completely flat and not move at all. I had two CT scans and a lumbar puncture which showed nothing.

I was discharged again and whilst I was in the discharge lounge still feeling extremely poorly, I felt sick and collapsed, unconscious, in the toilet cubicle. I was re-admitted and again I continued to suffer these extreme headaches. The following day I had a complete blackout. I have seen ENT doctors, a neurologist and cardiologist but they are all baffled.

Two weeks on I have had a few slight headaches but nothing major. As a result of a 24 hour ECG I have been referred to the cardiology dept. for a tilt test and an echocardiogram. Whilst in hospital I asked if it could have occurred due to hormonal imbalance due to the hysterectomy but they all said they don't know.

Recovery After Total Abdominal Hysterectomy, Vicki

Hi, my name is Vicki and I am 44 years old. I had a TAH on the 17th September, so I am six weeks and two days into my recovery. The reason for my TAH was like so many women the discovery of a very large fibroid. I'm not sure of the exact size of it but my incision had to be vertical due to the size of the fibroid. When I was first told I was having this operation I felt a real sense of loss and a part of me felt like a failure as a 'woman', apparently this is quite normal so if you feel this you are not alone.

I really wanted to let people know that I feel absolutely fine after the op; yes I have taken it easy and still am to a certain degree. I have been able to drive from four weeks, at first I only did little journeys but have not built it up so I can get out and about as the boredom of been stuck at home was driving me crazy. I have taken all the medical advice given to me but more importantly I have listened to my own body, it has a way of telling you if you have done too much.

So if you have been told the news that you need to have the op, please don't be scared, hopefully like me you will be well on the way to recovery within six weeks.

I really hope this may help some people put their minds at rest before they have this operation.

When Angels Catch Us, Madeleine Dunlop

I had been troubled by menstrual problems most of my adult life and had seven pregnancies in total, but unfortunately three of these ended in miscarriages. I always felt blessed in the four healthy children that I eventually had, even though those pregnancies too had also been difficult and not without their individual health scares. I knew my family was complete but even so, I could never contemplate getting sterilised, as I needed that security of still having the option available to us to have another child if and when the time was right.

The longing to have another baby never left me and many times over the years I had been relieved and disappointed that I had the birth control coil fitted as this took the decision and responsibility for my actions away from me. That all consuming urge to try again for another baby would at times be so overpowering, which if I'm truthful was usually fuelled as a result of one too many red wines of an evening.

My poor long suffering husband Paul would have given me the world but even he would caution me on the possible problems and health risks of having another pregnancy and was very much of the mind that we should be thankful for what we have.

I could not consider egg donation as the little baby would still be a part of me. But I had often said that I would gladly carry a baby in my oven for a couple who, for whatever reason, could not have a baby, as long as it was not genetically mine. I truly meant this and it's with regret now that I didn't explore this avenue further.

In August of 2006 I began to have more severe menstrual pain than normal and instead of the pain lessening after the period was over it had in fact gotten worse and I continued to have breakthrough bleeding. This was indeed unusual and although I would have been crippled during mid month with ovulation pain. I now found this was with me constantly. I struggled on until mid September and I eventually went to see a female doctor who advised me to get an urgent scan and as the waiting list, even for an urgent scan was 12 weeks, she had asked me to consider a private consultation. Paul and I were going on holiday the following Saturday so I made an appointment with the gynaecologist for the week I was due home. I confided in my sister the following day at a wedding of a close friend and tried to explain how frustrating and debilitating this condition had become, but I was naively hopeful it was a routine gynae problem, which could be easily fixed.

This planned holiday was to be our first trip away from the kids, apart from the rare night here and there over the years. A full week away for just Paul and me on a Mediterranean cruise liner was sheer luxury to celebrate our 15th wedding anniversary. I have to say this was the holiday of a lifetime and we enjoyed each other's company so well that it was truly the 2nd honeymoon that any happily married couple could wish for.

We fell in love all over again on that magical cruise and it was so refreshing and relaxing to do what you wanted, when you wanted without having to worry about the kids having enough activities to be entertained. We talked to them daily on the phone and emailed them each night with our adventures on board. This eased any guilt I had at going away without them. We enjoyed the company of two good friends whom we had gone on the trip with and made many new friends. It was a truly fantastic and unique experience, especially for a couple who had chosen to live their lives and spare time around the needs of their children. It was liberating and reclaimed us as a couple.

Although I was in a lot of pain every day, I took pain killers to combat this, even though as a rule I would be very against taking medication.

Hindsight is a wonderful thing and if we had known what was in store for us in the few short months ahead I truly think Paul and I would have gotten off that ship and stayed in that idyllic setting of Portofino, an island off the coast of Italy and hit the pause button on our lives.

I attended the consultation when I came back and a close friend accompanied me and was present when the doctor, after having scanned me and undertaken a full examination, gave me the unexpected and devastating news that I had what appeared to be a huge cyst on my left ovary filled with endometriosis which had also caused damage to my womb. A full hysterectomy was the recommended medical procedure advisable. I sat in his office and attempted to absorb the news and whilst I was naturally relieved to know that he didn't think it was cancerous I still had huge difficulty in coming to terms with what I had to face, no more children.

Coming home and exploring the options with Paul and our eldest daughter Laura the decision sounded so easy and non-negotiable. My health was at risk and the likelihood of having another baby at my ripe age was neither really feasible nor practical and wasn't I so lucky that this problem could be dealt with so effectively with surgery, which although major would be ultimately be for the greater good.

Common sense told me that this was the sensible option but what no one really understood was the overpowering sadness I was feeling, like a long jagged knife was twisting and turning in my heart. The acute realisation hit me that I would never again be able to experience the joy of being pregnant, never again be able to feel our babies kicking inside of me, never again having that one-on-one intimacy with your unborn baby, stroking your increasingly enlarged belly and no more would I experience that deeply personal communication that only a mother and her precious unborn baby within her womb can share.

This is the exclusive private world where fierce protective instincts and deep maternal love truly began for me and to a certain degree you want your precious baby to stay in that little protected cocoon forever.

Then of course nothing of any value can compare to the ultimate prize, the exquisite pleasure of being handed your new-born after an almost certain painful delivery and know this was truly the bestest feeling in the entire world.

I knew with such clarity that I would never ever feel whole again!

The consultant had written to my GP and had requested that she remove the birth control coil in case in some way it was inflaming my condition. She was very reluctant to do this as my pelvic areas were still so very tender and sore and also it was not a recommended time in my monthly cycle. An appointment was arranged for the following week, Wednesday 25th October 2006, as a suitable date to remove this intrauterine device and meanwhile I got a date for my hysterectomy operation for 8th December.

I telephoned my consultant's secretary to ask if the removal of the coil was absolutely necessary and she asked me if I was prepared to take a cancellation to which I readily agreed as my scheduled date would have left me very indisposed over the busy Christmas period.

Unbelievably the secretary rang back with a cancellation for the following Wednesday, the same day as I was due to get the coil removed by my GP. I remember thinking 'this is a strange coincidence'.

I was filled with such fear going into hospital that week and was in awe that it was three weeks to the day that I had gone for my private consult with my gynaecologist, and now here I was on the day of my operation. 'Too much, too soon', were the thoughts going through my head. I had already cried a river of tears for the 'no more babies' but now I was gripped with a paralysing fear as to what degree of pain I was to expect and what was the physical aftermath of the operation going to be like. I just wanted it to be over and I can honestly say that the waiting is definitely the worst part. I was inundated with text messages of support and I remember thinking this was something that I didn't want to undergo but had no choice in the matter, and if any of these well wishers were truly genuine they would take my place for the operation, or at least offer!

By this stage I had done thorough research on the condition of endometriosis and was armed with this new found knowledge that should help me make any decisions necessary. The control freak that I am didn't want to be baffled with medical jargon. I had a pre-op chat with my wonderful gynaecologist who assured me that he would not be, in my words, too scissor happy and would preserve my right ovary if possible to prevent me going into an early change of life. Counting the overhead lights on the corridor ceilings as I was being wheeled on a trolley on the way to theatre became very important to my sanity.

I was unable to joke with the porters as we bumped into walls and lift doors and the inevitable woman driver jokes and just wished and prayed it would all just happen quickly or, not at all.

I knew I had to stay calm for another while longer and then hopefully I would be so zonked I wouldn't care what was happening anymore. The nurse had just given me a pre-op sedative to help to relax me but it hadn't had time to take effect yet, or maybe I was just too anxious for any pill to calm me down.

Entering the bright lights of the operating theatre and seeing all the machines and staff dressed in their blue scrubs and confirming yet again my name, address, date of birth and my understanding of what procedure I was going to have was just so surreal. I could hear the whispered tones of junior staff being very sombre and respectful in the background. Was this for my benefit or was this in case they got a telling off from the big chiefs who were busy scrubbing up at the sinks?

The surgeons were laughing at some private joke and I remember thinking I was going to be at their medical mercy for the next few hours and my private inners and outers would be exposed to all and sundry present in that room. The reality of this ordeal suddenly just became too much for me and then, just as I felt that I was going to cry, I became blissfully aware of a wonderful floating feeling, I was there in body but definitely not in mind. Perhaps I was having the out of body experience I had read so much about! It was in fact the pre-op sedative starting to chill me out at last – if only I had been given that magic pill sooner.

Counting backwards from 10 was a welcome release…

I heard a lovely calm voice in my fuzzy head calling my name repeatedly coaxing me to open my eyes and I knew the operation was over and I thankfully I had come out of the anaesthetic successfully. Relief flooded my entire body until suddenly I was filled with a burning sensation in my lower abdomen. The owner of that motherly soothing voice belonged to a caring theatre nurse who then gave me additional pain relief by means of a syringe drive and the journey back to the ward was just a drug filled haze which ended with me slipping into a welcome sleep safe in the knowledge the whole operation was not as bad as I had expected.

I woke up and was vaguely aware of my husband Paul sitting patiently beside me, holding my hand, and remember feeling so so sorry for him as it must have been very sad and difficult for him to watch his loved one so out of it. I kept pressing the little button on the syringe drive and was convinced that no pain relief was to be got from it. After Paul left I tried to go back to sleep but the pain was getting progressively worse and I asked the nurse if I could get something stronger for the pain as this device was clearly not working properly. She was unable to give me anything as I had not been prescribed anything else and to compound matters the machine set off a loud bleeping sound every few minutes all through the night.

Not only was I in excruciating pain, no-one else in this busy ward could get to sleep either because of this alarm, except for another hysterectomy patient who was blissfully sleeping with the aid of a pain killing injection that I also needed but couldn't get. The morphine was supposed to be infused continually through this malfunctioning stupid syringe drive.

I don't think I have ever felt such self-pity as much as I did during that long, lonely, pain-filled night through into the morning when the cheery day staff came on shift. Thankfully one of the nurses was able to turn off the bleeping alarm and hastily agreed that I was in need of different pain relief and would get this sorted quickly.

My gynaecologist came to see me within a short time and explained to me that I didn't have the endometriosis condition that he had previously thought. What I had in fact was a large abscess growing on my left ovary which had attached itself to the wall of my bowel and the root of this was embedded round the birth control coil in my womb. He explained that a bowel surgeon was called to assist in my operation to remove this safely and he was confident that we had a successful result. He also explained that this abscess could have burst at any time and the consequences of this happening would have been fatal due to the poison, which would have instantly travelled into my bloodstream. A sample had gone for tests?

I absorbed this information as best I could but could not help thinking that had I not got that cancellation for the operation on the very day my GP was due to remove the coil I would not be here today. By removing the coil she would have inadvertently broke the root of this abscess and this would have resulted in my death.

What stopped this from happening? Why did I get a cancellation for that very day? Was this sheer luck or angel guidance from a higher level?

I truly believe that Divine Intervention by means of God's helpers, guided me to go to see that consultant privately and an inner voice urged me to ring up his secretary, which resulted in me having my operation on that fateful day.

'One can change one's fate but not one's destiny'

It was probably too soon to soon to come out of hospital that Tuesday morning but it was Halloween and I wanted the kids to enjoy their fireworks display and not have to worry about me not being there for them. They had organised a sleepover and I knew my Paul would be stressed to the hilt at having to deal with six noisy kids and the inevitable madness that is normality in our house, never mind me not being there.

One of the conditions to being allowed home was the patient had to have proper use of bodily functions and I knew this was going to be difficult as constipation was always a problem for me, especially after an anaesthetic. In order to pass this condition I took a hefty dose of Laxoberal laxative the previous night, which I was certain, would give the necessary result. By mid morning I still had no urge to go so I reluctantly asked the nurse for another spoonful of this sickly sweet medicine and lo and behold I performed the task in question admirably but with major stomach cramps.

As soon as the doctor had finished his rounds and I had assured him I was feeling tickety-boo and the rumbling in the jungle was indeed confirmation that the bowels were in motion, I phoned Paul to come and collect me, to take me home as soon as possible.

I only paid lip service to the strict instructions from the ward sister to the do's and don'ts of doing little or no household chores for the next six months. I thought this won't really apply to me as I'll be grand after a few weeks and anyway I avoided looking at her because she would know that I was not well enough to go home. If only I hadn't taken that extra spoonful of Laxoberal. I was crippled with excruciating stomach pain.

We packed my incredibly many belongings from the ward with lightening speed and even though I was feeling very peculiar, we set off like a bat out of hell out of there. We got into the lift which was on the way up but at least it was en-route to freedom. I felt so dizzy and weak but Paul was carrying so much stuff that he had no arms left to catch me when I nearly passed out in the lift. A man standing behind me had obviously seen my swaying and caught me just in time. The lift had stopped at a floor and the kind man tried to encourage me to sit down on a chair for a moment. Alas the lift had stopped at the very same floor from where we had just escaped from, so hell would have frozen over before I was getting out there to be recaptured. We got to the ground floor and I duly sat down and willed the dizziness to stop. Paul brought the car to the front door and I was free. I vividly remembered with despair all the happier times we had left this hospital with our precious cargo of a brand new baby on board and now we're taking the same trip home with an empty space inside me where my baby oven used to be!

The journey home was horrendous, as Paul seemed to have picked a shortcut that involved the most speed ramps in the whole of the city. I kept thinking my inners were going to fall out in the footwell of the jeep so it was with such relief that we arrived to the safety of home. Our son Rhys helped me down from the jeep and I allowed him to take my weight, as I didn't trust my wobbly legs to carry me safely inside.

My 85 year old mum arrived and once again was tasked with looking after the Dunlop's. I felt really ill and weak but at least I could watch the Halloween festivities from my comfortable recliner chair.

Over the next few days I began to feel so much better and was feeling guilty at my wee mammy busying herself with cooking and cleaning and fussing over me with the energy of a woman 40 years younger. She greeted all my friends and visitors with her wonderful warm hospitality and her wicked sense of humour. She was amazed at the amount of get well cards and floral bouquets that seemed to arrive on a daily basis and I too relished in the nurturing love that I was receiving from her and the good wishes from others. I was so grateful that our children were able to have their granny all to themselves and when she regaled them with stories from days gone by I too listened attentively and was filled with such admiration for this wonderful lady that I was so privileged to call my mum.

On Tuesday 7th November, exactly one week since I came out of hospital, my niece and her little baby came up from home to see me and I was so very touched at how she and many of the younger members of our family had visited, phoned or texted. We persuaded Martina, my niece, to stay until Laura and Auntie Ann arrived in the evening and we all sat down to a wonderful home cooked meal that mammy had prepared.

Wow! Two Years Post Op And I'm Feeling Better Than Ever! Jess 35 TVH

A bold statement indeed but a truthful one.

Two years ago aged 33 I was a ball of nerves bouncing around waiting to have my surgery. I was worried that my recovery wouldn't go to plan and the pain that would be involved. You know what? My recovery was steady, uneventful and a lot less painful than expected. Fantastic!

Yes, I had times when I felt like my tummy had gone ten rounds in a boxing ring but having a positive attitude and being well informed were my best forms of post surgery medication.

One year post op I felt really well but two years post op and I feel like a whole new person. Don't believe those helpful doctors who say that you will be fully recovered in six months. I feel one hundred times better than I did six months post surgery. Note: Interestingly these 'helpful doctors' have all been men .. mmm.. What do men know?!

I'm now getting used to my new found feelings of liberation and freedom after 15 years of misery and feeling like I was serving a bodily imposed jail sentence. In all honesty it's still taking some getting used to because I can't believe I'm so free of all the problems that used to have to be accommodated into my daily routine!

I am freer, happier and considerably better off financially!

I kept my two little ovarian friends and I can report that they are still up and running and ticking away very nicely indeed.

Oh and in case you were wondering everything else is working as it should. Make of that what you will ladies; it's our little secret!

There was a time when I couldn't believe I would ever stop thinking about having undergone a hysterectomy on a daily basis. Now I can go weeks with only a casual nod to the life changing experience that has lead me to be able to lead a much fuller, richer life.

After, Yvonne's Final Instalment

In October 2013 it will be six years since I had my operation. No regrets. Not one. At my four week check up I announced to my gynaecologist that I'd take that operation over PMS any day. It's six years now and I stand by that comment.

Initial recovery is slow, so accept it and try to enjoy it. Preparing the domestics beforehand, getting a cleaner, finding someone to change the bedding weekly and take towels and bedding away to be washed are all valuable steps and ones that both my husband and I appreciated in the aftermath. Getting back on your feet is important, but it is a big operation and really you should think of the full recovery as being a several year process. For instance, I struggled with the bed changing for nearly a year and couldn't carry much for nearly two years.

For me, the most difficult part of the process has been understanding my energy levels. I've never been stable - swinging between unable to move to being manic. That's PMS! I thought that manic was more normal, it was certainly productive. But my energy-normal is disappointingly low. But I'm in my 40s, healthy, and the last few years have been absolutely marvellous!

If you're scared, look through the actual operation day like it's a window; it's literally just a day. See the bigger picture. I felt like my life started for real in October 2007 and I have tears in my eyes just thinking of all the years of misery and pain I'd endured before getting to that point. If only I could have done it ten years earlier.

Good luck!

Glossary

101 Book - 101 Handy Hints for a Happy Hysterectomy

1B1/2 - Severity measurement of cancer in the tissues of the cervix

A&E - Accident and Emergency (hospital)

Ablation - A medical procedure that removes the lining of the uterus

Adenomyosis - A condition where endometrial tissue is found moves into the outer walls of the uterus

Adhesions - Fibrous bands that form between tissues and organs usually due to injury or surgery

Anaemia - Iron deficiency

Atypia - Structural abnormality in a cell

Bilateral Salpingo Oophorectomy - Removal of both fallopian tubes and ovaries

Bloods - Blood tests

BSO - Bilateral Salpingo Oophorectomy

BP - Blood Pressure

CA125 - A blood test for cancer screening

Catheter - Drains and collect urine from the bladder

CBT - Cognitive Behavioural Therapy (talking therapy)

CIN3 - Cervical Intra-epithelial Neoplasia 3 is high grade abnormal cell changes

CO2 Gas - Carbon dioxide gas used to inflate the abdomen

Coil - Mirena coil

Colposcopy - Examination of the surface of the cervix with a magnifier (colposcope)

C-Section - Surgical removal of a baby from the womb

D&C - Dilatation and curettage removes tissue from the lining of the womb.

da Vinci - Minimally invasive surgery using robotics

Dermoid Cyst - An overgrowth of normal, non-cancerous tissue in an unusual location

DH - Dear Husband

Done Couch - Women who have had a hysterectomy

ECG - Electrocardiogram measures the electrical activity of the heart

Embolisation - Non surgical treatment for fibroids that blocks off the arteries

Embolism - Blood clot, fat globule or bubble of gas in the bloodstream

Endocrine Problems - Disorders of the endocrine system, causing hormone excess or deficiency

Endocrinologist - A specialist that diagnose and treats endocrine problems

Endometrial Hyperplasia - excess numbers of endometrial cells, or inner lining of the womb

Endometriosis - A condition where cells from the lining of the womb appear outside womb

ENT - Ear, nose and throat

Epidural - An injection in the back to numb the lower body

Episiotomy - A cut between the vagina and anus during labour

ER - Emergency Room (hospital)

EUA - Examination Under Anaesthetic

FAB - Full Abdominal Hysterectomy

Fibroids - Non-cancerous tumours growing in or on the womb

GP - General Practitioner (general doctor)

Gynae/Gynaecologist - A medical professional specialising in women's health

HA - Hysterectomy Association

Haematologist - Specialists in blood disorders

Haematoma - A collection of blood usually within the tissue

HB - Haemoglobin is the protein in red blood cells that carries oxygen

HDU - High Dependency Unit

HRT - Hormone Replacement Therapy

Hyperplasia - Increased cell production in a normal tissue or organ

Hysterectomy - The removal of the womb (uterus)

Hysteroscopy - Inspection of the uterine cavity by surgical telescope

ICU - Intensive Care Unit (Hospital)

In Situ - In the same place

Intrauterine Device - a form of birth control inserted into the womb

IUI - Intrauterine Insemination treats infertility

Knife Cone Biopsy - Surgery that removes a sample of abnormal tissue from the cervix

Laparoscopic Hysterectomy - Keyhole hysterectomy

Laparoscopy - An operation which allows a surgeon to view the abdomen through a camera

Laser Ablation - Removal of the lining of the womb with a laser beam

LAVH - Laparoscopic Assisted Vaginal Hysterectomy

Locum - Temporary doctor

MA - Microwave Ablation

Macmillan Nurses - Specialist cancer nurses

Microwave Ablation - Removal of the lining of the womb with microwave heat

Mirena Device/Coil - A contraceptive inserted into the vagina for up to five years

MRI Scan - Magnetic Resonance Imaging

MRSA - Methicillin-Resistant Staphylococcus Aureus (infection)

Myomectomy - Surgical removal of fibroids

NHS - National Health Service

Norovirus - Nausea followed by vomiting and diarrhoea (infection)

OBGYN - Slang term for gynaecologist

Omental Biopsy - A sample of the omentum taken for examination

Omentum - A large piece of tissue that lies near to the womb

Oncologist - A specialist cancer doctor

Oncology - Science dealing with cancer and tumours

Ovarian Cyst - A fluid-filled sac that develops on one or more ovaries

Pain Bomb - Pain relief

PCA - Patient Controlled Analgesia

PCOS - Polycystic Ovary Syndrome

Peri-Menopausal - Pre Menopausal

Peritoneal Washing - A procedure used to look for malignant cells

Pessary - Used to support the uterus, vagina, bladder, or rectum

PET Scan - Positron Emission Tomography produces 3-dimensional, colour images

Phased Return - A return to work that gradually builds up the number of hours over time

Placenta Praevia - Low lying placenta that may block the baby's way out

Polycystic Ovaries - A condition where the egg isn't released from the ovary but stays on it forming a cyst

Polyp - Small growths

Progesterone - Female sex hormone produced in the second half of the menstrual cycle

Prolapse - A condition where internal organs fall out of their usual place

Prozac - An antidepressant

Pulmonary Embolism - A blockage of the main artery of the lung or one of its branches

Radical Hysterectomy - Removal of the womb, cervix, upper vagina and parametrium

Radical Surgical Resection - Surgery that removes the blood supply and lymph system supplying an organ along with the organ

RH - Radical Hysterectomy

Ring Pessary - A device inserted into the vagina to support the uterus, vagina, bladder or rectum

Septic - Overwhelming infection in the body

Spinal Tap - Anaesthetic through the spine (epidural)

SSP - Statutory Sick Pay

Statutory Sick Pay - Basic sick pay for employees (UK)

Subserosal Fibroid - Fibroids that develop on the outside of the womb

TAH - Total Abdominal Hysterectomy

TAH/BSO - Total Hysterectomy with Bilateral Salpingo Oophorectomy

TENS Machine - Transcutaneous Electrical Nerve Stimulation (alternative to pain killers)

Thrombosis - The formation of a blood clot inside a blood vessel

Total Hysterectomy - Removes the womb and cervix

TVH - Total Vaginal Hysterectomy

TVTO - Tension free Vaginal Tape Obturator

Urine Retention - The inability to urinate

Uterine Biopsy - Sample of the lining of the womb

Uterosacral Ligaments - A ligament that extends from the cervix to the back pelvic wall

Uterus - Womb

UTI - Urinary Tract Infection

VH - Vaginal Hysterectomy

Vaginal Hysterectomy - Hysterectomy performed through the vagina

Waiting Room - Women waiting for a hysterectomy

Womb - Uterus

Stories Listed By Subject

Not all of the stories can be categorised as contributors haven't said why they had surgery or what type of surgery they have had. The stories below can be categorised and the same stories may appear in more than one category.

Abdominal Hysterectomy

Adenomyosis

Cancer

da Vinci Hysterectomy

Heavy Bleeding

Laparoscopically Assisted Hysterectomy

Book Excerpt

I'd like to share an extract from one of our other books with you. 101 Handy Hints for a Happy Hysterectomy is exactly what it say's it is; hints and tips to help you prepare, undergo and recover from a hysterectomy as easily as possible.

"My own hysterectomy took place when I was thirty two; it changed my life. Before it, I was constantly ill, had serious problems with both endometriosis and IBS (irritable bowel syndrome) and would spend days every month in extreme pain. After it, I was suddenly well and I have never looked back, even though I couldn't have children.

But, I didn't know then, what I know now. I didn't know about the weight gain, the possible side effects of HRT, how tired I would be after the operation, when I could go back to work, what exercise I should (and shouldn't) do, and how much I would suffer from water retention. There were so many things I needed to know, but didn't and there were so many things I could have done to make my recovery easier, but didn't. What has always surprised me though is that even today, twelve years on; I'm still being asked these same questions by the thousands of women that contact The Hysterectomy Association every year. 101 Handy Hints for a Happy Hysterectomy was written to answer this need and hopefully it will provide you with some answers to the most common and frequently asked questions; as well as giving you some hints on how to make your recovery a successful one.

These hints are not designed to give you all of the information that is available; they are designed simply to raise your awareness so that you can then find out more about those things that matter. They are not in any particular order, although they are loosely divided into five sections: preparing for hysterectomy, getting ready to go into hospital, now you're in hospital, recovery at home and long term health. I would recommend reading through the whole book once and highlighting those that you might like to go back to later on. I would like to say thank you to everyone that has had a part in creating this book and mostly to the women that have contributed to the knowledge it contains, through their hints and tips for making every hysterectomy a happy one.

8. Coping with Fear

At times like this it could be easy to be overcome by your fears; fears that often aren't talked about, or even admitted to, in many cases. But, it is surprising how much better you feel when you do confront the fears you have about your hysterectomy because it helps you put them into perspective.

So what are your fears? Writing them down and admitting the worst that you think can happen, can help you to prepare yourself physically, emotionally and mentally.

Try this exercise one day when you have an hour or two to yourself. Gather together paper and pens and put them on a side table; then sit in your favourite chair and close your eyes. Imagine yourself in a beautiful garden, see the plants and flowers, smell the scents, touch the petals and slowly feel your body relaxing. When you are fully relaxed open your eyes and think about the worst things that could happen as a result of your operation; write them down as they come into your mind and try not to analyse them before getting them down on paper.

Once you have written down as much as you can think of, close your eyes again, imagine the garden and slowly relax your body. When you feel relaxed, open your eyes and read through the list you have written down. Now think about what you can do to find out more about each of the things you have identified. This may involve talking to your GP, family and friends, it may involve a bit of research on the internet or at your local library. As you find out more information write it down, you will find that you feel more in control and the fears, although they may still be there, will become manageable and you will also find that you are less stressed, and a calmer person finds it easier to recover from a hysterectomy. Fear is often a fear of the unknown so banish the unknown with knowledge."

That's it for this little extract. If you'd like to get your own copy of this best selling book then you can do so from all the usual places, including our own website and Amazon.

Paperback: shop.hysterectomy-association.org.uk

Amazon UK: www.amazon.co.uk/dp/0953244539

Amazon US: www.amazon.com/dp/0953244539

About The Hysterectomy Association

The Hysterectomy Association is a social enterprise. It was created to provide impartial, timely and appropriate information and support to women who were facing a hysterectomy. The biggest concern that the majority of women have is that they haven't been given enough information to help them make an informed decision, unfortunately this position doesn't seem to be changing much.

Over the years, the Hysterectomy Association has changed beyond all expectation and it is now achieving what it hoped to in the early days, simply because use of the Internet has grown so incredibly over the last few years. All of the information we produce is available on our website. We are a member of the NCVO (National Council for Voluntary Organisations) and are bound by their codes of conduct.

Our income comes solely from the money that our users pay for books and other products that we sell. If you have found us helpful at all then we would really appreciate it if you bought something from us or even sent a donation. You may wish to stock and sell our books yourself. We are always looking for help and we have listed a number of our own suggestions that may interest you, however, we are always willing to hear other ideas if you have them. If you would like to find out more information about working with us then please do get in touch with us by email at info@hysterectomy-association.org.uk.

We are based in Dorset in the UK and you can find out more about the association through the following accounts:

- Website: hysterectomy-association.org.uk
- Facebook: facebook.com/HysterectomyUK
- Twitter: twitter.com/HysterectomyUK

LinkedIn: linkedin.com/company/the-hysterectomy-association

Other Books From The Hysterectomy Association Include:

- 101 Handy Hints for a Happy Hysterectomy
- Losing the Woman Within